INTO THE WAVES

POEMS AND OTHER WRITINGS

BY BEVERLY D. BLANCHARD

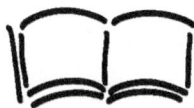

PB

Into The Waves : Poems and Other Writings
© Beverly Diana Blanchard 2012

Petra Books.
Ottawa Ontario Canada
613-294-2205 | petra@petrabooks.ca
petrabooks.ca

Library and Archives Canada Cataloguing in Publication
Blanchard, Beverly D.
Into the waves : poems and other writings
/ Beverly D. Blanchard.

Second print edition: black and white MAY 2012
ISBN 978-1-927032-05-3

First print edition: colour APRIL 2012
ISBN 978-1-927032-02-2

I. Title.
PS8603.L353I58 2012   C811'.6 C2012-900422-7

Digital format
ISBN 978-1-927032-04-6
PS8603.L353I58 2012   C811'.6 C2012-900423-5

Interior illustrations:
Quilt drawing (p. ii) and circles by Eryn Blanchard
Eagle sketch throughout, and *We are One, We are all Unique* (p. 62)
by Beverly D. Blanchard

cover: vangobot.com *Wave 11 Be Mine* by Luke Kelly

design: Petra Books www.petrabooks.ca

DEDICATION

To my brother, Steven.
All I can say is thanks.

Into The Waves

AUTHOR'S PREFACE

Is life just about struggle and work? Isn't there only one Earth that connects us all regardless of our nationality, religion or culture? These writings came about through a search for meaning. When I look at the waves on the ocean, I view them as being separate. But it seems to me that the waves are part of the whole ocean and there is no separation. Being part of the ocean provides me with a source of strength, confidence and happiness.

Although we are all connected, we are all unique. I offer these writings and drawings to you simply as my viewpoint.

bdb 2012

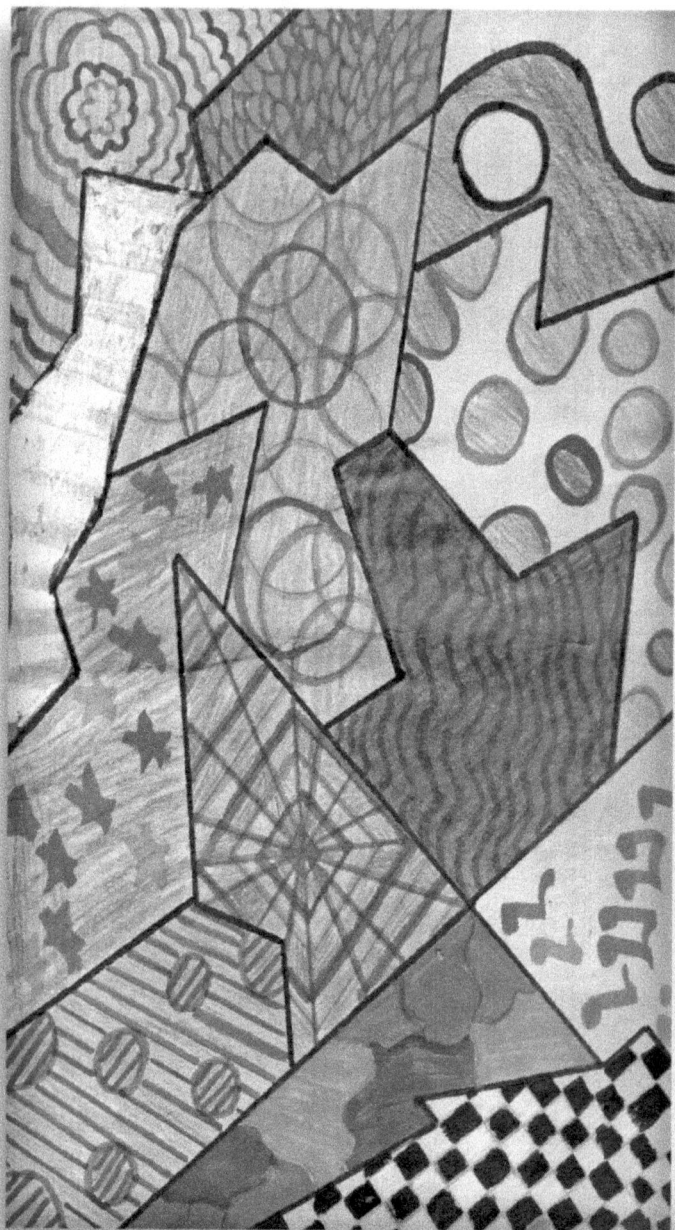

ACKNOWLEDGEMENTS

While there are too many people to recognize individually, there are a few people that I would like to acknowledge. It is to these individuals that I owe my heartfelt appreciation. Without their love, support and continual belief in my abilities, this book might still be in my head. I do hope they know how much they mean to me.

For their friendship, support and encouragement, Bob Finter, Luigia Cistera and Scott Cooper, who kept telling me this was worth doing.

Eryn, Scott and James Blanchard, thank you for unconditional love. To my mother, who in 2007 began her journey in the spirit world, I can only say that you were the best mother anyone could ask for and I was very proud to be your daughter.

Tom Tomlinson the Healer with the magic touch, thanks for fixing me and sending me back out to face the world with renewed hope.

Finally I would like to thank my designers and editors at Petra Books for making this book a reality.

facing page: *Quilt drawing* by Eryn Blanchard
from which the circles throughout are taken.

Into The Waves

CONTENTS

POEMS

OTHER WORKS

following page and throughout: *Eagle* by Beverly D. Blanchard;
circle from *Quilt drawing* (p ii) by Eryn Blanchard

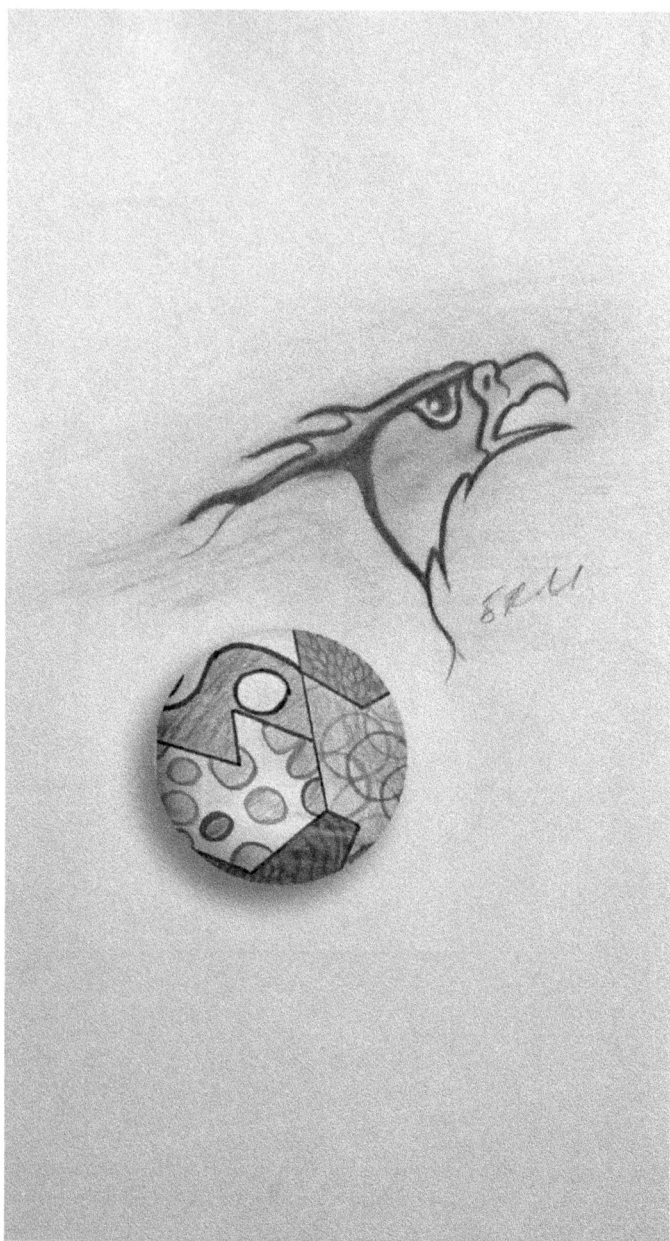

INNER SPACE

LIFE BEFORE BIRTH

It's warm in here.
I have no worries.
I have no doubts.
I have no fears.
Life is peaceful in here.
Warmed by a mother's voice and beating heart,
Each moment is eternal.
In the warmth of the womb I am at one.
I am free.
All is supplied.
Life is good.
Until that fateful day,
I enter the dark abyss.
My birth will become the death of my bliss.
The warmth of the womb will be no more.
My freedom will be no more.
Instead life will be limited by rules.
All designed to hinder my growth.
I will be given an identity,
and live a life judged by my material worth.
Can we reverse this birth?
Stay in this state of bliss.
For what awaits me is a world divided,
split and filled with contradictory spins.
It will never fit with my own true nature.

STEP

Step off the cliff.
'I can't.'
Trust.

She stepped forward,
and lifted her arms up to the sky.

'Should I fall head first,
or should I fly?'
Step off the cliff.

She stood frozen on the edge.
No magical wings unfolding.

Just do.

A moment of hesitation,
and she allowed herself to fall forward.
Only she didn't fly.
Instead she landed flat on her face,
and there she lay on the bridge.

I did say step.
'You could have told me there was a bridge.'
Would you have believed me?
'Probably not.'

She picked herself up.

'So, where are we?'
It is the bridge over the gap.

Cross over and you will know your true self.
'But I have a name and a job.
I know who I am.'

No, I am sorry to say.
You only know yourself as the wave.
Cross over the bridge,
and you will know yourself as the ocean.
'But in the ocean will I be free?'
Once a wave knows itself as the ocean,
how can it remember itself as a wave?
You become empowered by the whole.
Cross over the bridge and you will find bliss.
'What is bliss?'
It is living from the center of your being.
It is living from love.
It is your natural power.

'How long will it take me to cross over?'
The journey is not without challenges,
and there is no instant anything on the path.
You have work to do on yourself.
Do it joyfully, and the time is short.
Do it grudgingly,
and it will feel like eternity.

She knew once she took the step,
there was no turning back.
She would have to let go of the past.

'Will you be with me the whole journey?'
I have always been there.
It is unfortunate that you were not listening.
Instead you were focused on the ego,
which lead you down an illusionary path.

She stepped forward.
And life became serene.

DARK NIGHT OF THE SOUL

It's back.
The dark sinking feeling that your life is all wrong.
You've made the wrong turn,
and now can't seem to go on.
A series of questions spin round in your head,
Sometimes you think you are better off dead.
Doubt clouds your judgment.
Fear fills your head.
You think you aren't strong.
And really, as things stand;
how could you possibly go on?

Examining your life makes it all crystal clear.
According to society's standards,
your truths and beliefs must be based on fear.
For to survive here on Mother Earth,
you must see life as a curse.
Recognize it is always someone or something first.
You can't co-create life.
You were a fool to believe.
There is no power up your sleeve.
It was all a cosmic hoax.

Why look at your life, it's a joke.
Filled with lack,
at the present moment looks black.
You think you control life.
Well, that's a little green.
Let's just look at all the inconsistencies you've seen.

You live a world filled with darkness and fear.
There are the haves and have-nots,
and your white-lighter justice,
well, it doesn't rule here.
Greed gets ahead, and meanness prevails,
in this little world the Source Energy's love
is just a recipe that fails.

Hey, wait just a moment. a little voice said.
Look around. Raise your head.
The Creator's love is completely free.
All you must to do is open your heart and eyes to see.

Beauty abounds in all of creation.
You just have to believe.
Love of self is all you need.

A bright golden light begins to flicker within,
warmth melts the confusion
and you start to grin.
You step out of your fear to face life once more.

Assured of your future,
solid at the core.
For you have a right to be.
You deserve only the best.
As a spark of the Great Spirit,
You would not expect anything less.

REFLECTION IS JUST PROJECTION

Spare some change. the beggar chants.
You react with anger and sneer.
You would like to say,
'Get a job! I am having my own bad day.'
Or perhaps you look away,
and continue on your way.
Only to find much to your dismay,
Spare some change?
echoes out of every doorway.
Now your anger is really brewing.
It is getting quite hot.
For this very simple act of begging,
has now made you rage a lot.
All because a beggar crossed your path today?

What does this picture represent?
Could it be just a shadow of your own reality?
For they say everything is a projection.
Life is just one big mirror reflection,
reflecting what is going on deep within your own skin.
This anger is all about you.
This poor beggar committed no sin.
The situation is only an illusion.
manifested by you in an electromagnetic fusion.
For emotions bent on a negative slant,
simply reflect your own life reality.
So before you decide to condemn, be wise,
and check within.
For what resides on the outside,
only reflects the imbalance found inside.

Perhaps the beggar merely reflects,
the part of you that feels impoverished.
The part that begs to be fulfilled
through recognition from your boss;
a little more love from your spouse;
a little more wealth, fame or respect;
or perhaps the part of you that wants to be free.

Why do you beg for something you already have?
Find that part that feels some poverty or lack.
Turn the projector within,
and give your life script a new spin.
Readjust your movie screen,
And start filming those new scenes.
Let the inner space define your life.
Trust it, and you will have no strife.
Soon you will find there is no need to beg.
All is supplied.
In settling the illusion of the poverty within,
the outer poverty just fades away.

THE INNER GUIDE

In a world of complication and confusion,
trusting your inner guide can get rid of delusions.
One encounter is all you need.
Doesn't take much to plant the seed.

Leads you to a higher destiny.
Fills you with love for eternity.
Reconnecting can give you peace of mind.
Opens you to a relationship which is quite sublime.

It is the secret element in happiness,
and comes with a guarantee of absolute bliss.
A better friend is hard to find.
This is the most reliable kind.

It is always there, and does not interfere.
Just provides a few simple words, here and there.
And always does it with care.
It's interest: Your greatest good.

For your inner guide is the mighty *I am*.

NOT A TEST

In this life there are no road maps.
There are no grades to pass.
There is no one to tell us the future will be better.
No outside resources are necessary.

The source of your power lies within.
Yet we go on seeking answers from outside sources.
Never trusting our innate resources.
How foolish we are to think,
that if we pray real hard,
find the right angel or spirit guide,
the right dogma, religion or belief,
we will then follow the path of piousness.

Outside sources move us further away
from our energy source.
For all this time, deep within,
is a small still voice, just waiting to be heard.

Listen.
There is no better time.
Begin by stilling the voices of the mind.
Go to the level of no-nothingness.
Trust in the process.
Let the true voice speak.
There will only be bliss.

CUT THE MIND

Stop.
Watch.
Be still.
Be aware.
Listen.

Stop dragging yourself to the grave.
Stop repeating the same gestures,
and letting your mind drive you.

Drop your conscience,
and move out of the world of work.

Explore.
Avoid maps and guidelines,
and allow your heart to lead you.
With the innocence of a child,
allow yourself to experience the moment.

Learn to rely solely on yourself.
For a life of outside control is a life of convenience.
It is no life at all.
Instead it becomes slavery to a predetermined destiny,
in which you are told to accept your lot.
There is no bliss.
Instead there are only burdens and misery.
A life of misplaced happiness,
dependent on an outside world.

Yet all this time,
to achieve this one thing,
all one needs to do is turn within.
It is where life truly begins.

LET GO

Respond with totality.
Hold nothing back.
Recognize what could be done,
has been done,
and now be finished with it.
No regrets.
No guilt.
Just this moment,
in its perfection.

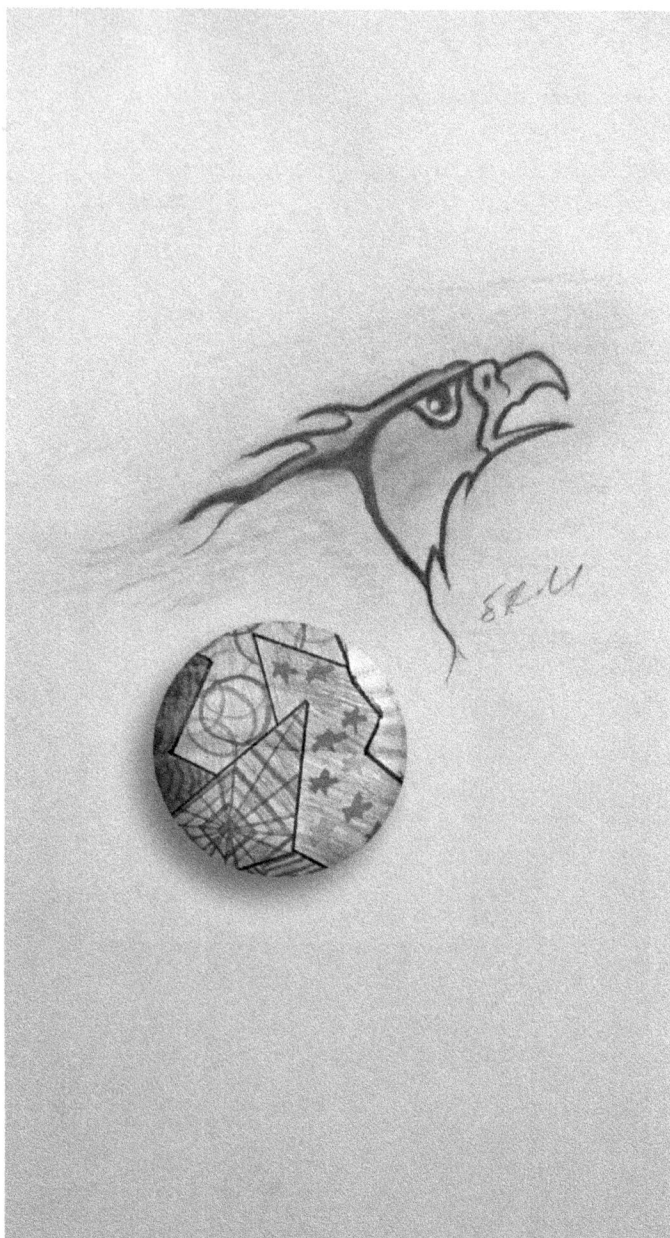

MANIFEST

YOUR RIGHTS IN LIFE

You have a right:

to the whole truth and nothing but the truth,
to breathe and take up space,
to be,
to trust yourself and your perceptions,
to a healthy life,
to abundance,
to love and be loved,
to be respected for who you are,
to have an opinion, and to be able to state it without fear,
to make mistakes, screw-up and get things wrong,
to dream big,
to say no without an explanation,
to show your true emotions and feelings without shame,
to expect only the best in life,
to work at a job that you love and earn a good income,
to have responsible and accountable government,
to choose your friends,
to happiness,
to be alive.

MY TRUTH

Nothing is guaranteed on my path.
But I face the challenge gladly knowing I grow.
My only loyalty is to truth.
My only consistency is to truth.
As I live,
I honor the spirit within.
I work in unison with the Source Energy.
I am a part of the whole.
I am the master of my destiny.
No organization confines me.
I belong to no society, culture or nation.
There is no protection in the crowd. That's only slavery.
I unleash my individuality.
Released from society's oppressive chains
of useless conditioning and repressive claims.
I am free.
I am a rebel.
Yet I fight against no one.
I embrace my own true nature.
I live my life, I live my truth.

CHOOSE

Pick a culture.
Any culture.
Any culture will do.
Only one though.

You can't be both.
Statistical purposes you know.
So the story goes.
Yet, I am a crossbreed.
Just what ancestry am I to believe?
I am not purely any culture, race or creed.
Just how am I to pick?
Knowing that deep within my DNA,
I am encoded with all my ancestors.
Tell me which little box do I tick?
These ways are contrary to my nature.
To define myself by this society's little box.
I must take from all worlds gone before.
For in doing so I maintain the balance.
I maintain the harmony.
I walk the oneness.
For one is not better than the other.
All my ancestors in this mixture are unique,
and I hold their memories,
their hopes, their loves and hates.
They are part me, yet they are not me.
I am a mixture of all those who have gone before.
Free to make my own choices,
and to know that the past is no more.
For I am here and the time is now.
I am all that I can become in this moment.
I am just me.
I am one with the whole.

Into The Waves

BE YOU

Society may want a carbon copy.
But look around.
There are no assembly lines.
There are only originals.
Look at nature.
No flower is ever the same.
Every tree is different.
Nothing in existence is duplicated.
And neither are you.
Everything in existence is unique,
and this includes you.

You are not a puppet, no one is pulling your strings.
At any moment, make the decision.
Drop the illusion you are powerless.
Drop the belief that to conform is correct.
Drop the program that you have no meaning,
or that existence is out to get you.
Existence is only for you.
Be innocent.
Be childlike.
Be trusting.
Be you.

Walk the fine line between madness and sanity.
For you were created as a unique being.
You are a shareholder in human consciousness,
and you have an important song to sing.
Find that song.
From the center of your being,
sing that song.
Sing it proudly.

Because without you the stars,
moon, sun, earth, sky and trees will miss you.
A small part of existence will be vacant.
Release yourself from the illusion of smallness.
Release your emotional hold on the past.
Remember, live in the head you live in stupidity.

Love opens the eyes.
Now is the only moment.
Here is the only space.
You are the only you.
Silence your mind.
Listen for that small, still voice within.
Live with an open and simple heart,
And, like a feather, goodness will find you.

NATURE'S SCHOOL

Truth can be found through nature.
There can be no conjecture.
It provides all the teachings,
casually demonstrates the natural order of things.
Watching it, man could find all his answers.
Destroy all this talk of life's cancers.
For within this world of the rational,
man has become one-dimensional.
He has painted his world in a deep gray,
and trampled a path through nature's lovely bouquet.
All done just to focus on the event of the day,
and day-by-day nature's messages go astray.
There is no stopping to smell those roses.
Man is commissioned with higher purpose.
There are more important things to do.
Like figure out who to screw.
To seek the truth one must turn to nature.
Let life be an adventure.

Be like water.
Move along like a drifter.
Always moves toward the depth.
It cannot be contained or kept.
Never hankers to be the first.
Does not think it is cursed.
It need not declare itself unique.
Nor does it shop at a certain boutique.
It does not struggle up a hill,
and never needs to take a pill.
It does not bother with consideration.
For it seeks balance in the destination.

Then there is the tree.
Among themselves they do not disagree.
They simply accept themselves as they are.
They never go bizarre.
They merely sway in the wind.
Do not see anything as sin.
They give of themselves unconditionally,
and live life quite peacefully.
They expect nothing in return,
never calculate how much they will earn.
Growth is not considered a horizontal line.
They do not operate with the word *mine*.

If only man would listen.
Nature would definitely enlighten.
Its messages are simple.
There is no need for any temple.
It is all around.
Through it, life's answers are all found.

LET BE

Take responsibility for your illusions.
You have created them.
Out of your beliefs you have created mountains,
filled with frustration.
You have lost the moment,
and built a life on future expectations.

Take back your moments.
Take back the now.
Lose expectations you have of yourself.
Lose the expectations you have of the world,
and of all the people in it.
Expectations can only lead to frustration,
and frustrations will always beat a path to misery.

For expectations are based on illusions,
designed to bring a life of disappointments.
Dissolve the expectation dilemma,
let go all expectations.
Be ruthless,
and then rest in the fullness of who you are now.

Let every situation be new and fresh.
Free from all past influence.
Accept who you are.
Let the silent watcher emerge.
Let go. Let be.
For what will be will always be.
There is no more.

MY LOYALTY

My loyalty is to truth.
My consistency is in truth.
I am not here to be famous.
I am not here for success.
I am not here for money.
If these things come to me along the way,
I am thankful.
My ultimate purpose for being on Mother Earth is truth.
Through truth I will come to understand
that I am a part of the whole.
I am the ocean instead of the wave.
Within this existence,
I am my own authority,
and the Great Spirit trusts me.

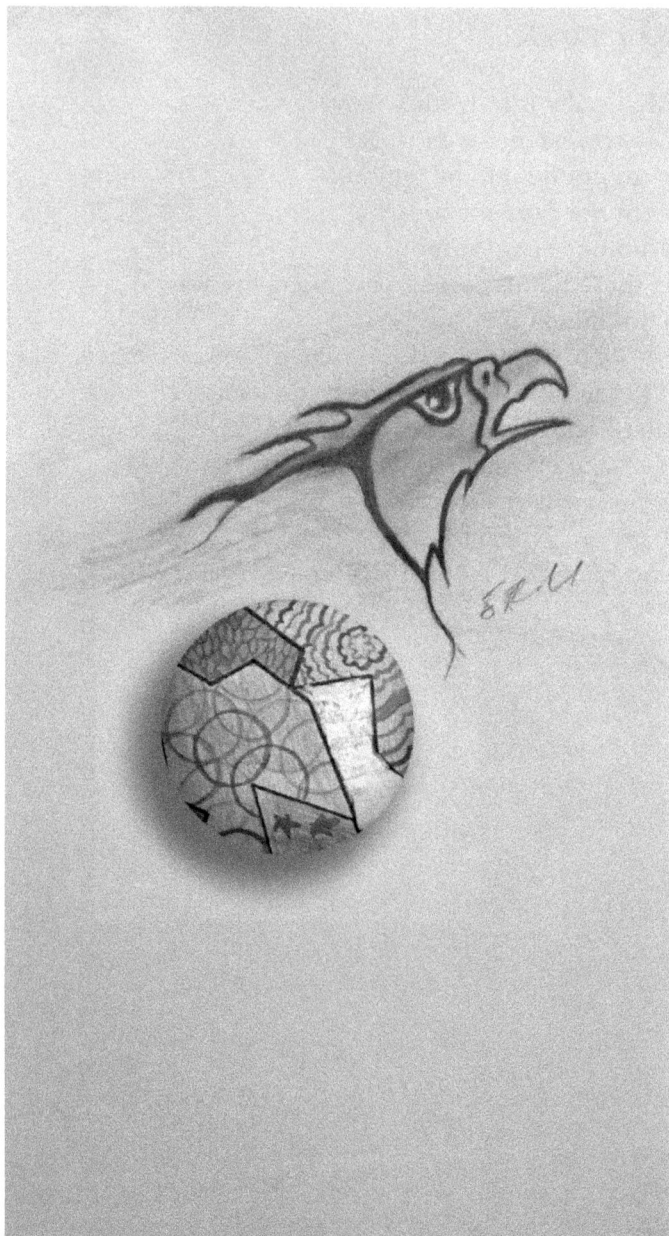

SOCIAL

THE RISING OF THE INNER SUN

Do not be afraid.
You have nothing to hide.
You have nothing to lose.
You need no one's approval.
There is no one to judge you.
So stop trying to be somebody.
You are already incomparably unique.
There is no need for improvements.
There is no need to add fame,
respectability, names and certificates.
In the end, they are all worthless.
For the more you try to be somebody,
the smaller you shall become.
The further you get from your true treasure.
The one that can be only be found within.
It is not what you have attained in the outer that counts.
It is only what is attained in the inner that matters.
It is only through the inner you reach new heights.
Give yourself permission to be.
Release all preconceived notions of what society expects.
Turn within and allow your true self to shine through.
When you finally do, happiness will burst forth.
The sun shall rise.
The flower will bloom.

THE CROWD

Man has become a crowd.
Divided.
Contradictory.
All split up.
Fragmented.
One moment loving,
and next, a monster
of epic proportions.
Man of many masks.
Defined by various labels.
Such a waste of energy.
He has chosen to live on the periphery,
the beggar's edge.
Where life flows against his true nature.
A life associated with struggle and lack.
Misery. The search for security.
Safety from the bogeyman.

Yet all this time the center remains untouched.
To touch it would prove man was an emperor,
a king of kings.
But no, man sits on the outer edge.
Caught in a schizophrenic state,
worrying about all the tomorrows.
Bamboozled by guilt-ridden pasts.
Who was I yesterday?
All the while,
wasting the present moment.
The one moment that will change the course of the day.

REFLECTING BACK

In hindsight, whatever I intended to happen in my life
went wrong.
Whatever I put my heart on was never attained.
The expected successes were met with disappointment.
My anticipated happiness never materialized.
Yet, through it all came that which I did not expect.
It turned out to be my greatest success.
An inevitable wellspring of joy
with not a single ounce of duress,
and all I had to do was move with the flow of Existence.
Instant joy was deployed.
Turned out, these were matters of great consequence.
It was at that point that life made sense.
It was not about some great purpose,
some achievement or prize.
It did not matter what legacy I left behind.
All that mattered was how I lived my life.
Were my actions based on love or hate?
To what part did I gravitate?

THE REALITY

They prepared me early,
for this journey called life.
Filled me full of facts and figures,
and taught me the basic rules of life.
Be kind unto others,
and always speak the truth.
Take responsibility for your actions;
a higher education will enhance all you do.
For this world of work was changing.
It was moving at lightning speed,
and the labour-market specialists,
claimed an educated workforce was all we would need.
To really succeed in this new economy,
all you needed was a university degree,
advertised with a lifetime guarantee.

So off I went to seek this university degree.
Spent four long years doing what-I-was-told-to-do.
All the while believing,
this education would prepare me for life's realities.
With it, I would be a true contributor to society.
I got that piece of paper, labeled a degree,
and figured I was now prepared for this adult reality.
So, off I went into the world of work,
armed with that degree,
naively assuming the doors would open magically.
But soon found out, the world of work was not the
book-reality.
Basic rules of life, given to me at birth, were all
ancient history.

For in this little world,
the rules were changed to fit the game.
Life was about working for corporate gain.
Politically correct was the name of the game,
and calling a spade a spade,
well, in this workforce,
was simply the wrong way.
Honesty and ethics became clever spins,
used by management to cover up sins.
Hiring was another strange case.
Facts do not necessarily matter.
The only qualifications are in the spin.

So, now here I sit on the edge of retiring from this scene.
Looking back, the world of work consumed my life,
and I became a casualty of mundane routines.

Get up.
Eat.
Work.
Eat.
Sleep.
Get up.
Repetitions of a daily schedule,
ho-hum actions that are locked into a life pattern,
of thirty or forty years.
All the while, I have been missing the point.
Ever so slowly it has been passing me by.
Seasons have come and gone,
and life has become just a blur of activities.
Memories of what might have been,
could have been, gone.
All blown up in smoke.

Into The Waves

Unless I wake up,
I will go on missing the point.
I will go on postponing the now for some future date,
a time when all conditions will be perfectly met.
When I will have enough money,
a bigger house, a better car.
I will have that promotion to enhance my security.
When everything is right,
I will then be able to live.
Only the time will never be right,
and all of this will be excuses for not following my heart.

Excuses that have brought me to this dead-end,
where I have realized,
happiness does not reside in the outside treasures.
For with all my material resources,
there still exists, deep within,
an emptiness, a hole which no outside illusion can fill.
Time to awaken from this grey slumber
before death takes me and turns me to dust.
For to stay on this path will mean
I will have settled for an old, dull routine.
I will die never quite understanding why I was here.
Instead I must turn within.
Discover who I am,
and why I walk on this Mother Earth.

So, I have taken to watching butterflies,
as they dart across my path.
In an erratic little fashion,
they teach me how to enjoy life.
When they arrive, my inner child arises.
I become enchanted with life again.
My inner being sings in indescribable ways.

Innocence is reborn.
If only for a moment,
I have no cares and worries.
I am no longer that little wave in the ocean.
I am one with all that is around me.
I am the ocean.

Treasuring butterflies,
and observing nature's work,
I have now taken to watching trees.
They are in abundance,
and there are so many for me to see.
My inner child is now playing constantly.
Watching the dance of nature has given me inner harmony.
Through nature existence shares its secrets with me,
and I have learned,
life is not as serious as we believe it to be.
I am free.

THE FOUNTAIN OF YOUTH

They searched high.
They searched low.
They took courses,
and bought magical potions.
They devised incantations,
and rituals.
When all else failed they took the surgical route.
Yet, still they found there was no fountain of youth.
It proved to be another cosmic joke.
There was actually no need to search.
The fountain of youth was not very far.
It was actually quite close.
It was found in your core.
The voice within that speaks so demure.
Ever so softly,
it awaits to be heard.

A DIRTY WORD

In our compact adult world,
play has become the dirtiest word.
We have become intoxicated with the word *work*.
It is an addiction with all sorts of motivations.
Mostly so we can buy an assortment of mundane things.
Live in castles like queens and kings.
Yet, the more we have, the less we hold,
and life does not unfold the way we are told.
At some point you soon discover,
it was shadows you were chasing all through your life.
Rushing for that money, prestige and power,
all just illusionary matters of mundane concerns.

Matters of great consequence you never savored.
There was never time to stop and smell the flowers.
Revel in their beauty. Become intoxicated with their
fragrance.
No time to play in the park, or just go for a walk.
Watch the butterflies flutter along.
Listen to a bird sing its song.
Take the time to visit some foreign land.
No, work always seemed to get in the way.
Matters of leisure were put away for faraway days.
Only faraway days never come.
Life becomes dependent on other things.
Simply put: working for a living.

Step off the path.
There is only now.
Play and dance in the light of the sun.

THE WORD JUNGLE

In this world, the use of words has become discretionary.
You cannot rely on the dictionary,
for it seems words are a lot of mumbo jumbo.
It now requires you to be a sleuth like Colombo.
Seems conversing has become like a rumble in the jungle.
Words, I am afraid are in an utter bungle.

They just don't have the same old meaning,
and depending on the user it can be downright deceiving.
For sometimes words are manipulated.
Then there is manner in which they are translated.
If the word and the action do not seem to comply,
somewhere there could be a little white lie.

Look at the words destiny and fate.
They now are words used to abdicate.
No need to find your path home.
Plead you are suffering from some syndrome.
Someone else is responsible for your actions.
Life is the result of the stars' reactions.

The word love has been casually cast around.
You wonder if it can actually be found.
It has become the opposite of what it was supposed to be.
Love is just no longer free.
It comes with strings and expectation.
Love today even comes with litigation.

The meaning of success has been flipped.
The whole of mankind seems to be pistol-whipped.
You are judged by what you possess.
That has become the meaning of success.

It doesn't matter about your true being.
It is all about your material wellbeing.

Free will has become a product of the ego.
It is now marketed as our *amigo*.
Yet, following it will bring you great misery.
There is no magic in its wizardry.
It will take you away from the original source.
Lead you down a dangerous course.

Words are tossed bogusly around every day.
Be careful about what you hear, think and say.
The power of words has been known throughout history.
Abracadabra, Alakazam and Hocus Pocus
are the keys to the mystery.
For each of them simply state,
With my word I create.

THE DRAG

Blind to roses, to butterflies,
no enjoyment in music,
no dance.
There is only a dragging
as the journey to the grave begins.
Questing for money,
a life of acquisitions,
accumulations,
hoarding.
Misers,
meaningless meanderings,
mundane routines,
day in, day out.
Society's graveyard defined as *life*,
end of the road - nothing but death,
at which point success
becomes failure turned-inside-out,
life now defined by the inner.

THE LIAR'S ROSEBUSH

The mirrors have shattered.
There is glass all around.
The fantasy was just another illusion.
Reality has no obligations.
The illusion can be no more.
The truth has been revealed
through a parting of the clouds.
A liar's rosebush had been concealed.
Flowering so cleverly,
and packaged so skillfully.
Yet, hidden beneath were dangerous thorns,
sharp and lethal they proved to be,
with flowers that bloomed so abundantly.

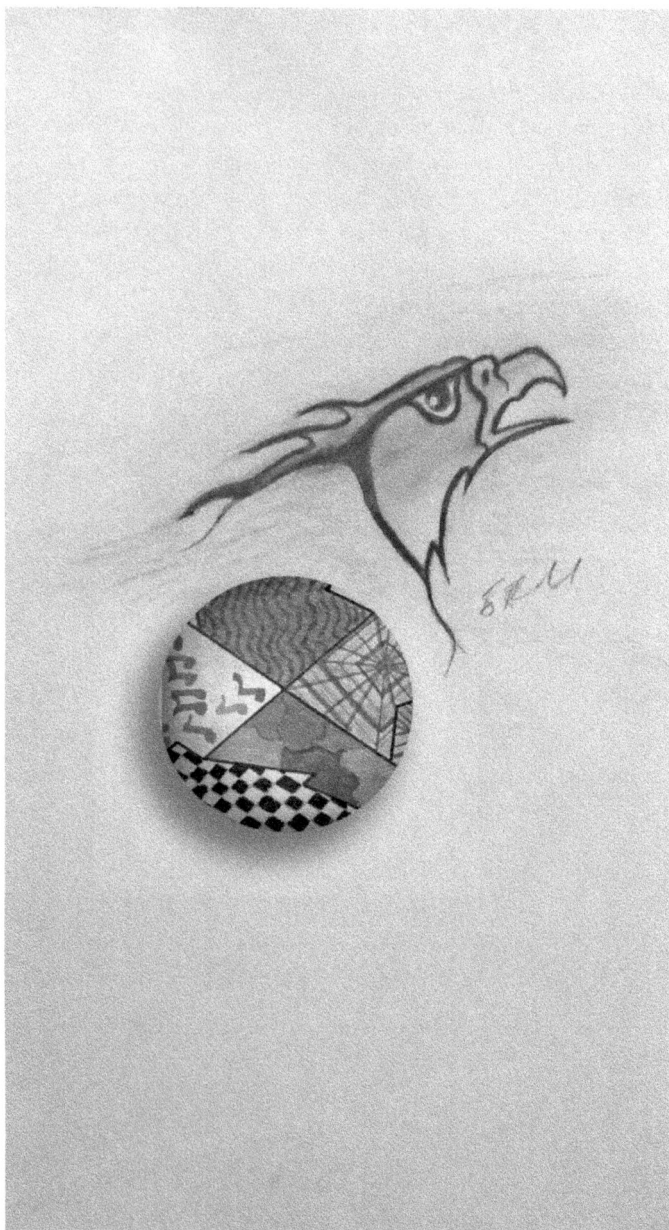

LOVE

JUST SAY GOOD-BYE

Love cannot be forced.
It is not dependent on laws or conventions.

The length of love is meaningless.
It may be an hour or a lifetime.

As long as love is the binding force,
It has meaning, it has depth.

When it has gone, be done with it.
Be thankful it has come your way.

Just say a simple good bye.

TWO MINDS, TWO HEARTS

In a debate between two minds,
truth is not significant.

It is not necessary.
Its whole game is a lie.

In a love between two hearts,
truth is always significant.
It is necessary.
It is the nourishing of the soul.

In the game of life it can be said.
Win a heart and you shall never be defeated.
Win a mind and you shall always have an enemy.
For the ego will always stir you to competition.
It is only through the heart you are truly free.

RELATIONSHIP CHANCES

Even if there is hate.
There is still a chance for relationship.
It is difficult, but hate can change to love.
If there is love,
there is a very good chance for relationship.
But beware,
just as hate can change to love,
love can also change to hate.
For love and hate are two sides of the same coin.

Then there is indifference.
There is no chance for a relationship in this state.
All chances end with indifference.
For indifference can never change to love, or hate.
Indifference is a lower range.

It is colder than cold.
It cuts deeper than deep.
No consciousness exists in its action.
No awareness.
No feeling.
Just a cold and calculating deed,
which knows no love or hate.
When indifference does arise,
no relationship can survive.
For neither love nor hate can penetrate.

COME DANCE

Be endlessly curious.
Let your mind wander.
Vow to learn something new.
Ask questions.
More questions.
Ask even more questions.
Don't take *because* for an answer.
Become childlike again.
But not childish.
Open to innocence.
Release yourself from past conditioning.
Release yourself from fear.
Let go of emotional attachments.
Let go of everyone's limiting beliefs.
Smile at strangers.
Smile at yourself.
Laugh.
Laugh often,
at yourself,
at the world.
Be mentally spontaneous.
Be carefree.
Live.
Live with abandon.
Dare to dance the dance of life.
Dare to be you.

THE GRANDEST LOVE AFFAIR

The greatest love affair comes not from someone else.
With the other there is bondage.
There is dependency.
To fall in love with another is nonetheless good.
But should you want the grandest affair of all,
all one must do is fall in love with the whole cosmos.
Dance to the universal symphony.
Let love beat within your heart.
Let appreciation consume you.
Let thankfulness become you.
Only then you shall experience the grandest love affair.

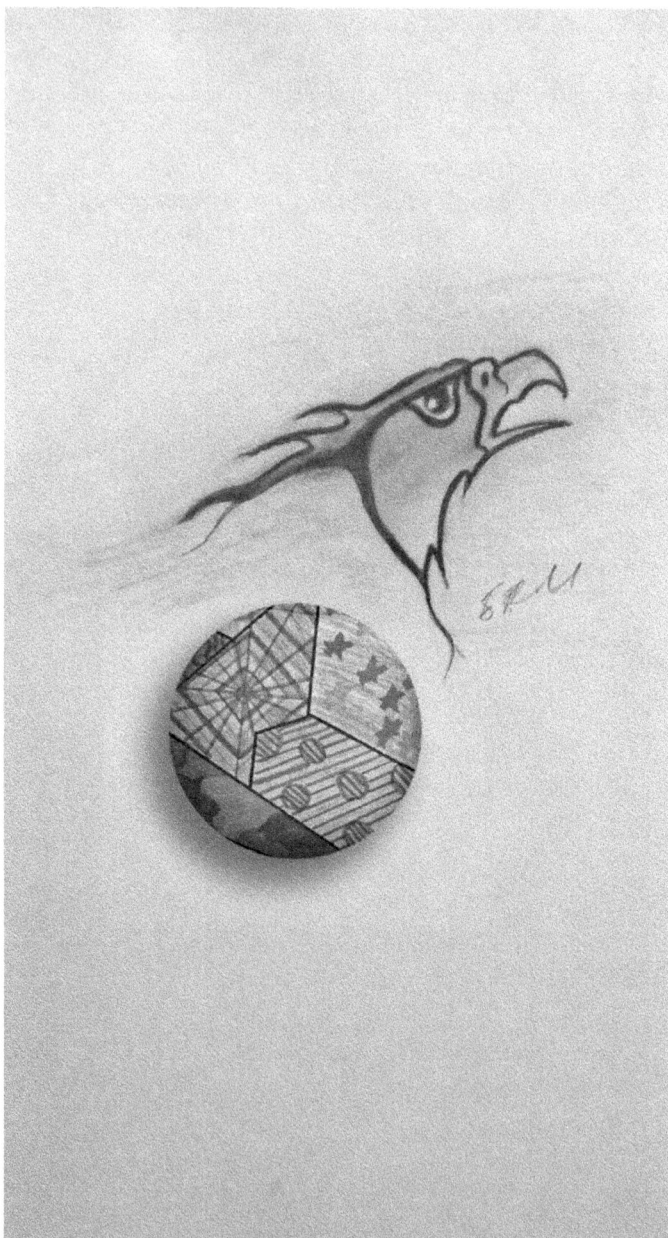

PSYCHE

THE VICTIM IDENTIFICATION GUIDE

Blame others.
Believe the world is out to get you.
Practice self-flagellation.
Abuse yourself verbally.
Tell yourself often, *you are good for nothing,*
and absolutely useless.
You are a bad person.
Make 'why me?' part of your everyday vocabulary.
Wallow in your misery.
Complain about everything.
Make excuses for everything.
Focus on what is wrong with your life.
Live in the past.
Worry about the future.
Make all your choices based on past experiences.
Choose not to live in the moment.
Expect the worst.
Think you are cursed.
Above it all, take no responsibility for your actions.

THE FINAL PICTURE SHOW

Say what you want.
Do what you will.
But remember:
Every action you take,
every word you recite
will come back to you haunt you on your final night.

For recorded in the cosmos is a file about you,
and nothing is forgotten, deleted or moved.
On that final night the movie will roll,
and there on the screen your life will unfold.
Every action you took and its resulting impact,
from the moment you were born,
to when you breathed your last.
The movie will end
and will await your review.
Out of ten stars, how did you do?
Did you spread good cheer?
Or was hate and fear your mantra here?

The final movie is really up to you.
It's actually your choice what you view.
One piece of advice I wish to impart.
Make your choices from love, and only from the heart.
In the end your movie will be filled with laughter,
and happiness will be yours to last.

LIFE'S LITTLE HOLES

After falling into one of life's little holes,
I figured I had learned to avoid them.
Anticipate them. Walk around them.
Until it happened again on one of those days,
I fell into the depths of hell.
Another of life's little dark holes.
Only this time a secret saw the light of day.
It was the reason why,
I still wavered between heaven and hell.
It came as a flash of insight,
that seemed to light up the night.
It was the solution to all of my problems.
With a simple change of mind,
my hell could become my heaven.

Flip a switch and my heaven would be my hell.
So the roots of all my anguish and misery,
were simply a result of me.
My life was my responsibility.
A simple change in perspective was required.
Just consciously watch where I put my thoughts.
Because when I act without awareness,
and get caught in life's dramas,
I inevitably fall into hell and land
down into those deep, dark cold holes.
However, if I act with full awareness,
and move along with the flow
I inevitably end up in heaven,
where there actually are no holes.
So it is how I use my consciousness,
that brings me to heaven and hell.

LIFE OF A CLOWN

Even if the whole world laughs at me,
I shall revel in my ordinariness.
My no-nothingness.
Knowing I danced, I sang, I played.
Lived the life of a clown,
without embarrassment,
all the while searching for the truth.
I can show you things to impress,
but the greatest of my treasures,
cannot be laid before you.
It is the source within me,
that connects me to the whole.
It is the source,
that provides all of life's understanding,
and is never demanding.

KEEPING UP FAÇADES

It is a world of illusion,
filled with collusion.
Nothing is really as it seems.
People don't say what they mean.
There are fake doors.
No real guarantors.
It is a tangled web of lies.
Somewhere they kissed the truth good-bye.
Abundance was to come with ties,
Based on a few simple lies.
In a world where everyone owes,
have we sunk to new lows?

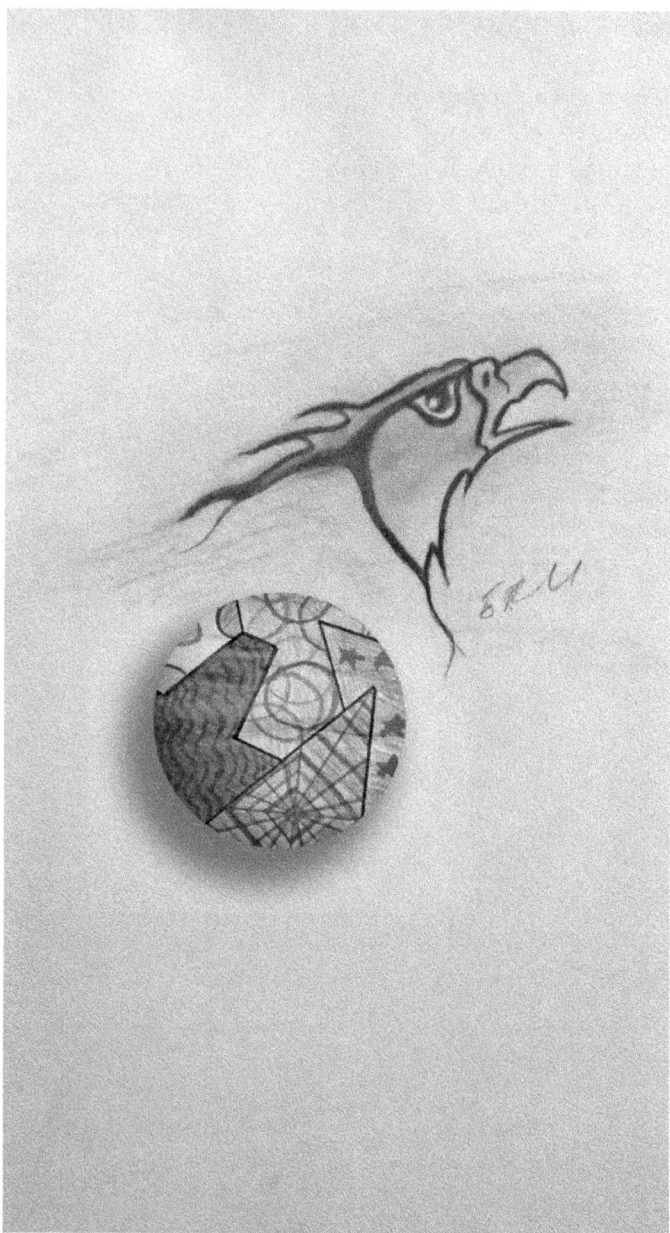

SONGS WITHOUT MUSIC

NO TOMORROW

Some day. One day.
Maybe. Tomorrow.
Next week. Next month.
Later. When I catch a minute.
Just one more thing to do.
Someday I will do it.

A million excuses.
A million lies.
More words uttered with no meaning.
Time passes.
Seasons change.
Time flies.

Life gets filled with the same old.
Same old faces. Same old scenes.
Mundane routines. Day-in, day-out.
Dragging myself to the grave.
For some demented belief.
Inherited at birth on this Earth.

Everything good was to be found upstream.
Life was meant to be a struggle.
The goal was hard to reach.
Society's little scheme.

AWAKEN

Awaken dear people, the choice draws near.
There is no reason to fear.
It is very clear.
Make the choice.
Only love here.

There is no threat in the light.
It is time to shine bright.
The darkness has fear.
Call it out of the closet, and it will not come near.
Where there is light, darkness cannot appear.

Remember — rosy illusions cannot stay.
As you discern what is real, all else will fade away.
Truth will shatter the illusions.
It will reveal the intricate delusions.
There will be no other conclusions.

Reach outside the box.
Expect the best, you will outwit that fox.
Drop the belief you have sinned.
See the Divine as living within.
Reconnect with your highest kin.

Be still, and know love is here.
There is nothing to fear.
Abundance is all around.
Waiting to be found.
Look past the mound.

When you listen to the voice of heart inside.
Expect life to become a magical ride.
Opportunities shall multiply.
Synchronicities the Universe shall supply.
Love is all you apply.

Awaken dear people, the choice is here.
Release all fear.
Love is here.

DON'T TALK ABOUT IT

Don't talk about it, they say.
It is just the old way.
It doesn't exist today.
Besides, people will just roll their eyes,
and think you are crazy and telling lies.

Don't talk about it they say.
It's best to let go of the old ways.
We are educated, intelligent beings today.
The old ways were just crammed with superstition.
Education taught us to let go of that magician.

Don't talk about it they say.
It is no longer part of our culture.
We have joined the new world vulture.
We have the feathers and drums
— what more do we need?
Forget the old ways, like talking to trees.

Don't talk about it they say.
The Europeans landed on our shores.
It was a time when we closed many doors.
We forgot about the power of our connection.
Instead caught up in worldly possessions.

Don't talk about it they say.
There is no talking with the trees.
There is no dialogue with the breeze.
The rocks do not sing with glee.
We do not have the power to just be.

Don't talk about it they say.
The old ways can't be used today.
It is all a reality of another day.
We are in the modern dream.
We can no longer drink from the old stream.

Talk about it I say.
It was a part of who we were,
before that fatal day.
Aligned with nature, moving with the flow.
Spirit was all around, life was a *deep let go*.

Talk about it I say.
We can bring back those powers
to help us today.
Spirit has always been around.
Quiet the mind — listen for that sound.

Talk about it I say.
Nature is asking us to come and play.
Unleash the power of our feeling,
and come to our greatest healing.
Talk about it I say.

THE CLEAN-UP

It is time.
Clean up the irritations.
Let go of petty frustrations.
Lay to rest your grievances.
Stop thinking of this or that.
Release yourself from past mistakes.
Recognize you had some aches.
Forgive yourself for anger and hate.
Do unto others where it really relates.
Relinquish your struggle to survive.
Allow yourself to come alive.
Just let loose, enjoy the ride.
Should at any point you have to surmise,
remember that Love is on your side.
Quiet the mind.
Go within.
There are several options with which you can begin.
The choice is yours.
Just pick a door. Go explore.
What are you waiting for?

A SIMPLE TRUTH ABOUT LIFE

It is really rather simple.
There isn't much to know.
Abundance is freely given,
— just accept the flow.

For life is meant for living.
Free from struggle and the blues.
Suffering is not a virtue,
and sacrifice you need not choose.

So let go of personal put-downs,
and recognize the truth within.
Life is about possibilities,
and endless opportunities to win.

For there are no real losses,
in this game of life, you see.
It's really about perspective,
and seeing it all positively.

THE WAIT

Death was knocking at his door.
Beckoning his spirit to come and soar.
We knew it was only a matter of time,
before his breathing would stop with one last chime.
He would then become the Father we once knew,
kept within our hearts, a fond memory to view.

We waited for his last breath.
We waited patiently.
Watching. Holding. Crying.
Afraid for his pain.
Afraid for our loss of a Father we loved.
A man who now lay powerless in a hospital bed.

We knew the final curtain call was near,
with celestial trumpets sounding in the air.
The time had come for our Father to open the door,
and cross that threshold to be in pain no more.
Death was waiting to bring him safely home,
where he would then retire from the usual human form.
For a celebration was now in the making,
and all who had gone before, were ever so happily
awaiting, the arrival of one more.

We waited for his last breath.
We waited patiently.
Watching. Holding. Crying.
Afraid for his pain.
Afraid for our loss of a Father we loved.
A man who now lay powerless in a hospital bed.

He breathed his last with his youngest son on that night,
and casually took his final walk into the light.
Where all who had gone before, greeted him with delight.
They cheered him on, they welcomed him home.
To a place where he would no longer moan.
For here in love, he was reborn.

The family left in silence on that cold November night.
The spirit of their Father had walked into the light.
And although they say he is happy and free of pain,
the family still feels numbness,
as though they were short-changed.
For no matter what was said.
Their beloved Father was now dead.

THE POWER

I've got the power.
I can make the darkness cower.
It didn't cost me any cash.
I learned it in a flash.

It was such a simple thing to do,
and was always taken kindly to.
Learned it when I was young,
a smile could always get you sprung.

For in that little smile,
was a simple power that made people go that extra mile.
Offered strangers a more pleasant day,
when they may have been dismayed.

So why not try this simple little trick?
You can learn it in a click.
Just turn up the corner of your lips.
Release the seriousness of life that grips.

See the beauty in it all;
and a smile will never become a wall.
Instead it will warm the day,
and bring light to darkness in the most mysterious way.

BE TRUE TO YOU

Know thyself the masters say.
But each little soul looks for the easy way.
Some grab onto the illusion of the day.
Living in fear is their way.
For some it becomes the material trappings,
life is about the gift wrappings.
Certificates or recognition hang on the wall,
but in the end they mean nothing at all.
For at the moment of death all your fictions disappear.
Naked you stand in front of the mirror.
Will there be a whole life wasted?
Was it all just manipulated?
Without all your possessions from this land,
where do you actually stand?
For the real treasure can be found within,
it is deep down beneath the skin.
Will it shine bright on that final day?

TREAD LIGHTLY

Tread lightly on Mother Earth,
for we have caused her significant hurt.
We have been insensitive to her needs.
Over the years we have left her to bleed.
And now we rape and pillage her more,
all to make that financial score.
No thought of the generations to come,
mankind can be quite dumb.
Never do consider her losses.
Even though, she carries all the crosses.
It's all about taking her resources,
extracting all of her rich sources.
What will we do when she can give no more;
when she angrily fires back a roar?

ODE TO A TREE

Oh, to be a tree.
What a luxury that would be.

For in the tree kingdom there is no jealousy.
There is no pretentious hypocrisy.
They are completely free.
They are allowed to just be.
They don't belong to any society.
They don't suffer from anxiety.
Unless of course man comes with an axe,
and then a tree suffers panic attacks.
Other than that they bend and go with the flow.

They gently grow upwards ever so slow.
There is no death in their life.
Life is not filled with strife.
They weather almost every storm, and never mourn.
Have no ambitions —no inhibitions.
They just accept themselves as they are.
They have no issues about house, job or car.
Life for a tree is just about being.
There is no striving, wheeling or dealing.

Oh to be a tree.
What an absolute joy that would be.

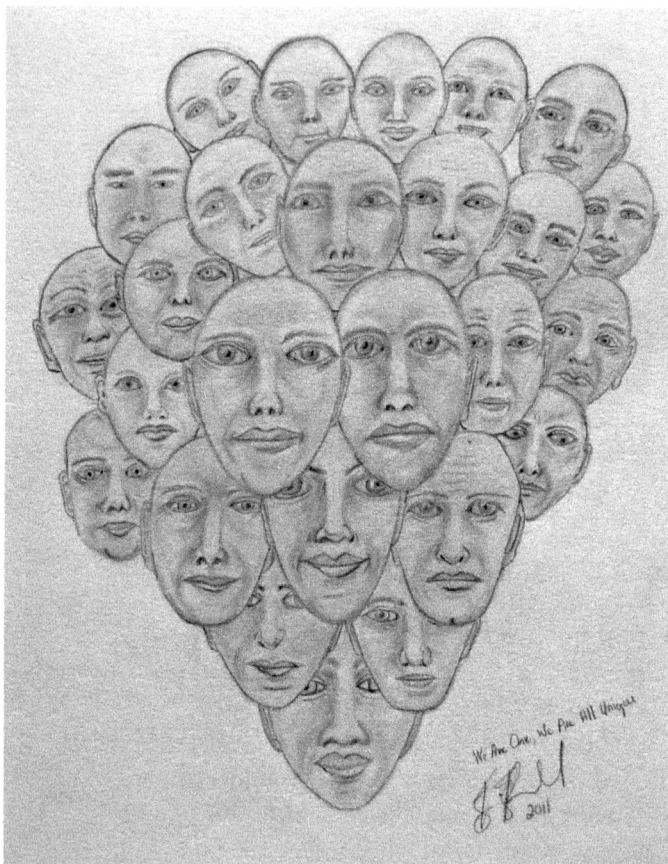

We are One, We are all Unique by Beverly D. Blanchard

THE SASSAGIS
(A PARABLE)

Once upon a time, a long, long time ago, things were much different on Mother Earth than they are today. Back then, there were no planes, trains or cars. There were no factories or stores. No electricity buzzing through wires. No computers or video games. No pizza delivery. No ATM bank machines. No one had to carry money or credit cards. There were no banks. There was only a community of spirits who saw no diversity and who understood the ancient laws of the Universe. During those days, Mother Earth was filled with tranquility. There was never any fighting and there were no bullies. All the inhabitants of Mother Earth saw each other as a spark of the Great Spirit in physical form; and it was in their best interests to get along with each other.

Since the spirits of yesteryear understood the ancient laws, they knew the importance of using their emotions as a personal guidance system. If something didn't feel right or good, they knew they were not aligned with the Great Spirit's energy. If something felt good they were aligned with the Great Spirit's energy. There was connection. Since everyone lived by the same law, life on Mother Earth was spent enjoying existence. Everyone looked for the best in everything and that which they focused upon came to them. Of course this was a long, long time ago.

They say that back then, Mother Earth was really stunning. She had the most lush, green forests which

63

housed the unicorns, elves, fairies, pixies, wolves, birds and other spirits. The air was always clear. The sweet smell of flowers filled the air, and sometimes the wonderful fragrance cast an unending spell of happiness on everyone on the land. Everyone played and worked together in complete joy and everywhere you looked, everyone was smiling because the more you smiled, the happier you became.

Not only was the land filled with an abundance of happiness. Long ago, there flowed a great network of crystal clear streams, rivers and lakes across the body of Mother Earth. These waters bustled with life, and flowed into oceans filled with mermaids, seahorses and dolphins who would always make their way to the shore to play with their friends who lived on the land amongst the tree spirits.

During that time Mother Earth was considered the most beautiful planet in the whole of the universe. She radiated so much loving light that many space travelers used her light to navigate the galaxies. It had also been said, that the reason she had so much beauty was in the legend about her creation. Many of the old Elders had said the Great Spirit had created Mother Earth as a gift for the Mother of all Creation. For the Great Spirit knew, without the Mother of all Creation he could never have created the universe. So in a gesture of thanks, he filled the planet Earth with all that was beautiful, and created a place where only love was to abide and bloom. Grandfather Sun's light provided warmth and protection for all of Mother Earth's children, and at night Grandma Moon would guide her oceans, and the Star People would shine their loving energy upon her to ensure the spirits inhabiting Mother Earth would always live in harmony. It was really a paradise back then. So after he created Earth, the Great Spirit gifted it to the Mother of Creation. Of course the Mother of Creation was overcome with emotion and she cried happy tears. He then dedicated Earth to the Mother of Creation by calling it Mother Earth.

Life on Mother Earth from that point onwards was about having fun. For all Mother Earth's children, every-day seemed like a vacation. That is not to say they did not work. They had a lot of things to attend to, however because they were passionate about what they contributed, they never considered it work. They considered it to be just like playing. Wake-up, pursue your passions and do what needs to be done. Everyone had a role. There were no worries or fears. No one worried about not being liked. Everyone considered everyone else as being incomparably unique. For on Mother Earth everyone knew they looked different but it did not matter. No one cared. For each of them knew, they were all family. Everyone knew they were a spark of the Great Spirit, and everything they needed would always be provided for them. Provided of course, if what they wanted harmed no one or thing. All they had to do was ask and trust that sometimes what they wanted would come through pathways they had not considered. They also knew that they could not force the manifestation of their desires. For under the Law of Allowing they understood that when they focused too hard on what they wanted they pushed it away. So sometimes it was best to ask and then detach from their request.

Well as you can see, in those days, life on Mother Earth was quite first-class. Happiness filled the air. Everyone was accepted as they were which meant that there was never any fighting on Mother Earth. In fact, the word fighting did not even exist. If there ever was a problem, and they always looked at problems as challenges, the solution was always for the good of the whole. Love had the final say. They would actually ask, *What would love do?* In asking this one question, they always discovered the answer.

It came to pass that things changed with the arrival of the evil ones, known in Ojibway as the Sassagis, to Mother Earth. With the Sassagis love would not be considered. The Sassagis were known throughout the Universe as the evil mean-ones, and the night they arrived, well let us just say, Mother Earth lost a lot of her light. Things would never be the same. The old ancient laws got forgotten. The Spirits of Mother Earth forgot who they were and started believing the propaganda and stories of the Sassagis.

It all started one fateful night long ago. You see the Sassagis lived out on the outskirts of the Universe and had been put there because they were a part of the Great Spirit that he had not been too thrilled about. He actually created their own planet, and because of their propensity to unscrupulous living they had caused much damage to their own planet. Anyway the Sassagis had heard about Mother Earth and being the greedy spirits that they were, made their way to reap some of the benefits of the most beautiful planet in the universe. So on that fateful night a long, long time ago, the Sassagis landed on Mother Earth. It had been a long and difficult journey for the Sassagis, but they were a very determined bunch, and somehow, no one will ever understand how, they arrived on Mother Earth. Since they had been traveling a long, long time, and had stopped in at a few other planets on their way, they had gotten in the custom of arriving in the darkness of the night. They certainly caused a great uproar on Mother Earth with their night time arrival. The people on Mother Earth had never felt anything like it. It was worse than an earthquake. The clamor of the Sassagis' club-like feet pounding on Mother Earth shook the ones who lived on land from their beds, and it rippled out to the oceans creating a tsunami that whipped the mermaids, seahorses and dolphins out of their beds. It was the first time the people on Mother Earth had ever felt fear, and it would not be the last.

Now, let me tell you a little bit about the Sassagis. They were ghastly looking ogres with personalities that matched their looks. They had two stubby horns that stuck out of their heads, and a black eye sat in the middle of their forehead. It would eerily roam from side to side. Their noses were smudged into their faces, and they had a permanent snarl painted across their lips. Even if they tried they would never be able to smile. Their bodies were covered with long strands of dirty, black hair, and little bugs shaped like dollar signs flittered about them. They were not very graceful. You certainly would not see them in dance class. Their monstrous hairy club feet lumbered out in front of them as they marched along snorting and spitting green pools of slime. It was said, *Where the Sassagis goes, nothing grows.* It was true. Many of the planets they visited on their journey to Mother Earth had suffered irreparable damage, and now all that was beautiful on Mother Earth was threatened. Where the Sassagis went everything was flattened and trampled, and sealed with green slime which hardened and blackened with time.

To add injury to insult, the Sassagis were not kind beings. Actually, they were downright miserable and mean. Oh sure in the beginning they were a friendly bunch but as time went on they changed. Their true colours began to surface and they started taking over everything. They took over the land and houses. They began telling the original inhabitants of Mother Earth what they were to believe. They were actually very mean and did not believe in love or kindness. Their only concern was collecting these strange little pieces of paper which, they stated, were the official currency of Mother Earth. Some say the reason for their meanness was the small size of their hearts. They had big heads but small hearts which meant they could not be all that lovable.

Well one of the ways the Sassagis loved to get their way was by using fear, and the more the people of Mother Earth feared them, the more power they ceded to the Sassagis. Knowing this only made the Sassagis use fear even more. They would continually taunt and bully the poor people of Mother Earth. The Sassagis also believed that it was alright to trample all the forests, and throw garbage in the waters. They believed the people of Mother Earth were indebted to them for their arrival. They really liked things to be gloomy. In the darkness of the evening, they would merrily stomp through the flower patches and lush forests spitting globs of their green slime which hardened and blackened with time. And as each day went by Mother Earth got darker and sadder.

Trying always to come from their hearts, the people of Mother Earth tried in vain to respect the Sassagis' ways, but the more they tried, the worse things got. The people tried to be friends with them, but the Sassagis were not interested in sharing or being friends. *All for me.* was the Sassagis' motto. They were only interested in taking over Mother Earth, and making her look like their homeland way out in space. That homeland was void of color, and being so miserable all the time made their planet a really sad place. They actually liked it that way, but they had also heard about Mother Earth's treasures and beauty, and they wanted to find out if the stories were true. Could there actually be a planet filled with so much love?

So, the more the people of Mother Earth tried to be friends with the Sassagis, the more the Sassagis bullied them. Bullying was something the people of Mother Earth had never come across. Things were supposed to be settled through love not through anger and meanness. Yet, the more the Sassagis bullied, the more fear filled the air, and since the Sassagis liked using fear, the more powerful they became. As time went on, the people of Mother Earth started hiding in their homes, and, seeing an opportunity, the Sassagis moved in to take control of things.

They began making lots of rules, and giving lots of orders. One of their first rules was that all meetings should be held at midnight. You see, the Sassagis never liked the light of Grandfather Sun. Some say, it was because Grandfather Sun melted some of their meanness. The meetings were never fun and usually ended with the Sassagis spitting green slime everywhere. Some of Mother Earth's people did attend the meetings for a while, but they ended up agreeing with the things the Sassagis had decreed just because they were afraid. The Sassagis always made it a point of intimidating the people, and since many of the people were a lot smaller, they always backed down. They forgot about the power they had within.

It was most unfortunate that all the people of Mother Earth stopped going to those meetings, because, one morning they awoke to discover that the Sassagis had posted a whole new set of rules on the trees.

NOTICE TO THE CITIZENS
OF MOTHER EARTH

WE THE SASSAGIS, RULERS OF MOTHER EARTH DO HEREBY DECREE THE FOLLOWING RULES TO ALL THE CITIZENS:

1: NO MORE SMILING OR LAUGHING FROM EIGHT O'CLOCK IN THE MORNING TO SIX O'CLOCK IN THE EVENING.

2: NO GOING OUT IN GRANDFATHER SUN'S LIGHT UNTIL AFTER FOUR O'CLOCK.

3: NO SINGING.

THERE WILL BE PUNISHMENT FOR ANY CITIZEN WHO BREAKS THESE RULES.

SIGNED, THE SASSAGIS

Life was no longer filled with happiness for all of the people of Mother Earth. Instead, they lived in constant fear that the Sassagis would hurt them. They also began to doubt themselves. As ridiculous as they knew the rules to be, as citizens they followed them. They stopped smiling and laughing. They forgot about their power. Instead, they started worrying about how they were going to avoid the Sassagis. They were living in fear that the Sassagis might hurt them. There was so much fear about the Sassagis that whenever they were out with others, they would spend all their time talking about how scared they were of the Sassagis.

Well, they say that if you think about or talk about something long enough it will come to pass. So, with the citizens of Mother Earth continually talking about their fears, the Sassagis did indeed start to hurt the citizens of Mother Earth. They started issuing harsher punishments to anyone who broke their rules. Bullies do those sorts of things, and because no one will stand up to them, they get away with it. Many of the fairies had their wings pulled off losing much of their power. Some of the mermaids had their hair cut off, and becoming prisoners of the land. The unicorns were also met with ruthless punishments. Many had their horns ripped right off their heads. Everyone was so consumed with fear that they began hiding in their homes.

Happiness had turned to sadness on Mother Earth. Rainbows no longer filled Father Sky. Dark clouds blocked out Grandfather Sun's light. The flowers had all been trampled to the ground, and gone were the fresh smells of flowers that had filled the air. The lush forests were no more and became open spaces of cindered trees. The waters were filled with trash. Everything was covered with green slime that hardened and blackened with time. With laughter and happiness outlawed, and their environment destroyed, the citizens of Mother Earth were forced to move into cold, concrete cities. With no light from Grandfather Sun, the days got colder and everyday and in everyway, the light around Mother Earth got darker and darker.

Well, the Great Spirit was watching how things on Mother Earth were progressing, and he was not very pleased. He was not happy that the Sassagis had made their way to Mother Earth. It was not part of his original plan. He had created a planet specifically for them, and he had thought since he had put it far out at the edge of the universe, they would never find their way to Mother Earth. He was wrong. The Sassagis never did listen to the Great Spirit. Always did what they wanted without any consideration of their actions. They proved to be the dark side always set on destroying things.

Now as the Great Spirit looked down upon Mother Earth he felt a deep sadness. His gift to the Mother of Creation was slowly being destroyed and he really had no idea what he was going to do. He also could not let the Mother of Creation know what was going on. It would break her heart. He had to think of something to do and he had to come up with an idea fast. The Sassagis had destroyed much of Mother Earth, and as much as he wanted to swoop down and punish them, he knew he could not. You see, a long, long time ago when the spirits were still young, they complained to the Great Spirit that they did not have enough freedom to be themselves. The

Great Spirit had suspected that the Sassagis had put the rest of the spirits up to it, but, he decided to take it under consideration. So, he thought about it for quite some time, and decided he would give all the spirits 'free will' to make their own choices without his interference. So now with the situation such that it was on Mother Earth, the Great Spirit could not intervene directly. The spirits all had 'free will', and they could make choices about their situations. He could however do something indirectly to get the people of Mother Earth to stop thinking about that which they feared. For as long as they allowed the Sassagis to have their way with fear, they would take advantage of the people of Mother Earth. The Great Spirit sat back and thought about the situation. How was he going to get the people of Mother Earth to change their thinking?

He thought about it for what seemed to be a long time. He could not exactly meddle in the situation directly. He had given his word to all the spirits, and 'free will' was working well on the other planets. How was he going to do this without interfering? He came upon an ingenious idea. He could send some reinforcements to remind the people of Mother Earth of their power. That way he would not be interfering directly. With that he summoned into his Great Hall, some of his Angels, Wise Ones, High Priestesses, Sorcerers, Wizards, Shamans, Star People, Grand Masters and Witches. They sat around the grand circular table for what seemed like two Earth years. You see, in the world of spirit there is really no such thing as time.

After much debate, it was decided that an advance team of Angels would go to Mother Earth to remind the people that they were safe and protected, and to let go of their fear, doubt and worry. Since the Wise Ones, Grand Masters, Star People and Wizards were such great change-of-shape artists; they would mingle with the people of Mother Earth and help them remember the power in their thinking. They would also start breaking all of the Sassagis' ridiculous rules. The first to go would be the no smiling or laughter. The team of Sorcerers, Witches and Shamans would work together to develop a spell to cancel the damage done to Mother Earth by the Sassagis and restore her to her initial beauty. They would also find a potion and spell to not only vanquish and send the Sassagis back to their planet but they would bind them to that planet. No simple task. If the potion and spell were off in the slightest, there could be negative consequences for generations. The Great Spirit's team had their work cut out for them.

So after much preparation, the Great Spirit's team set off to complete their parts of the plan to restore Mother Earth. Within days, the citizens of Mother Earth started whispering about seeing and hearing angels. Angels that were telling them to change their focus away from fear since it all starts with a change in thinking. The citizens of Mother Earth got really excited, but since happiness and smiling were outlawed by the Sassagis they hid their excitement. They swallowed their smiles. Should the Sassagis find out about the Angels, they would be most upset, and when they were really upset, they were downright mean and nasty.

Well time went by on Mother Earth, and on the surface of things, superficially, not much really changed. The citizens on Mother Earth tried to change their thinking and it worked a bit but then there were setbacks and they lost some of their optimism. It had been centuries that all this had been going on, and they were feeling rather downtrodden and hopeless. Everyday they wished the Sassagis would not bother them, and everyday their wishes did not come true. They were beginning to think the Angels had abandoned them, and they were alone in this battle. The citizens of Mother Earth were so busy worrying about being hurt by the Sassagis, most did not notice the new citizens moving in around them. Until it happened on one fateful afternoon when some of the new neighbors were heard laughing and singing out on the streets at two o'clock in the afternoon. The sound of laughter echoed off the concrete walls and made it sound like there were thousands of citizens singing and laughing.

Now, it had been years since anyone had heard the sweet sound of laughter on Mother Earth, and the sound caused quite a commotion. No one really knew what to do. The laughter was such engaging music to the ears of the citizens of Mother Earth. But they knew what might happen if they joined into the laughter and singing. The Sassagis might find them and put them into the gloomy, black dungeons they had built. Anyone who disobeyed the rules ended up there, and they were not pleasant. There was no freedom anymore on Mother Earth. By all accounts if you were in the concrete cities or dungeons, you were still in prison. Yet the sound of that laughter and singing brought strong stirrings in their hearts.

Well the sweet, sound of laughter vibrated out, and could not help but stir in the hearts of the citizens of Mother Earth. Many started to smile, but, when they heard the thunderous sounds of the Sassagis clumsy feet lumbering toward the sound of the laughter, they quickly wiped the smiles off their faces. Once again they swallowed their smiles. The smiles may have been off their faces, but inside they felt a warm glow in their heart, as they heard the repeated whisperings of the Angels telling them to trust and let go. At this point, many of the citizens of Mother Earth started to come out of their homes. As they peered up into Father Sky, a small crack of light pierced through the gray clouds. After centuries of living under this gloom, Grandfather Sun was melting away the darkness. The citizens of Mother Earth knew it was time to take back the Earth.

In the meantime, the Sassagis were running toward the sound of the laughter and singing. The sound of the laughter was not music to their ears. The song being sung was so grinding to the Sassagis. *Catch us if you can. Our song will never end. Catch us if you can. Ha! Ha! Ha! Our song will never end!* On and on and on it went. To the Sassagis it was like fingernails running down a chalkboard. They hated the sound of laughter and singing more than anything else in the universe. It sent shivers down their crooked spines, and made their dark hair stand on end. It was quite funny to see them in that shape. Well the Sassagis were having a terrible time trying to catch the elusive laughter and singing. It seemed that whenever they finally made it to where they thought the laughter and singing was coming from, they heard it from another place. The laughter and singing were moving at incredible speeds. Now, the Sassagis were not especially pleased about this, and could not understand what was going on.

Laughter and singing had been outlawed a long time ago. Now, hundreds of years later there was never-ending laughter and singing. They just could not understand where it could be coming from since there was no place to hide on Mother Earth. Under the Sassagis' rule, there were no more forests anymore. There was only blackened tar. After years of the Sassagis snorting green slime everywhere, not much grew on Mother Earth.

So, the Sassagis chased after the laughter for a long time. On and on the Sassagis ran. Almost looked like a dog chasing its tail. After some time, you could say the Sassagis became obsessed with the fleeing laughter, and like the citizens of Mother Earth, they forgot about the power of their thoughts. They kept telling themselves that some day, one day they would capture the laughter, and silence it. But it was never to be. Using the words 'someday' or 'one day' always results in nothing. It shall always mean tomorrow and there is no tomorrow. There is only today. So, the Sassagis chased the laughter and singing all over Mother Earth. They could not capture that laughter and song, because it was always two steps ahead of them singing:

Catch us if you can. Our song will never end. Catch us if you can. Ha! Ha! Ha! Our song will never end!

Meanwhile back at the concrete cities things were beginning to change. With the Sassagis' legions of armies off chasing the laughter, the citizens of Mother Earth began to enjoy some of their new found freedom. The Wise Ones, Grand Masters, Star People and Wizards that had come to live among them began persuading more and more of the people of Mother Earth to venture out beyond the walls of the cities. Slowly, the people of Mother Earth stepped through the gateway, and as each did, they discovered how much damage the Sassagis had done to the forests and waters of Mother Earth. There was lots of garbage strewn everywhere. Mother Earth looked worse than a garbage dump.

As the people of Mother Earth walked along the pathways leading out to what used to be the forests, they looked around in horror. Where once trees and flowers grew, there were only cindered trees and ashes. There was no colour. Mother Earth's majestic waters were filled with the Sassagis' green slime some of which, over time, had not yet fully hardened. As the people of Mother Earth looked around, a feeling of helplessness filled their beings. They had no idea where to begin to heal Mother Earth to her earlier beauty, or even if they could. Just as they started to cry, Grandfather Sun's light pierced through Father Sky revealing a tiny rainbow. It was a sign of hope for the people of Mother Earth.

Now as the people of Mother Earth were figuring out where to begin repairing things, the Sassagis' armies were still chasing after the laughter. They ran all over Mother Earth, and green slime was flying everywhere. After about ten times around Mother Earth, the Sassagis were quite exhausted, and very angry. Many of them just collapsed on the ground. It was now potion time. At that moment, the Great Spirit's team stepped out from behind a large curtain, and just as the Sassagis lunged at the team, the Sorcerers, Witches and Shamans swooped down and threw a vanquishing formula at the Sassagis, which would send them back to their planet for good.

With the Sassagis vanquished, the Sorcerers,

Witches and Shamans quickly formed a circle, and began to cast a magic spell to return Mother Earth to her previous beauty. There was only one problem. In their haste to cast their spell they did not notice that a few of the Sassagis had managed to remain behind. That was most unfortunate, since it weakened the power of the spell and only restored Mother Earth to 99% of her beauty.

Now the Great Spirit's team of reinforcements could have gone after those few Sassagis but after a bit of discussion it was decided to let them remain on Mother Earth. It was decided that because of 'free will' it was important that the people of Mother Earth see living examples of what they do not want to become.

Those few Sassagis reproduced and multiplied, as did all spirits. So that is why we have some mean, miserable people on Mother Earth today. They provide you with contrast and give the opportunity to see that you always have a choice. You have free will. You have the power to make your life miserable or happy. The power resides in your choice.

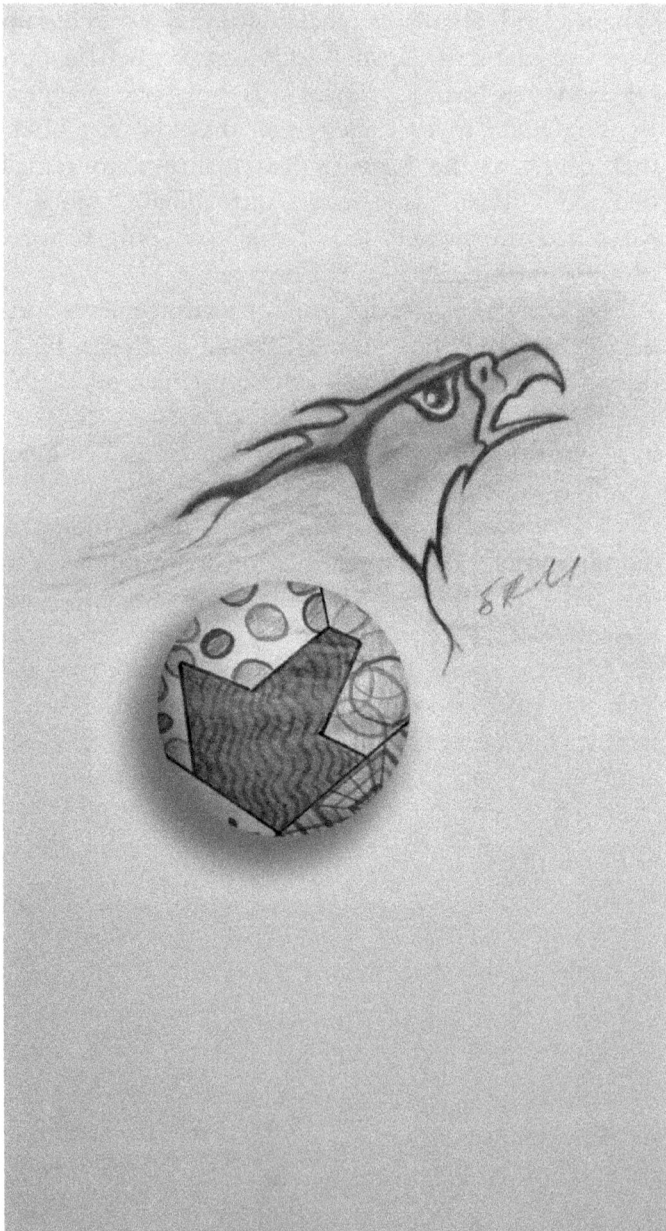

UNIVERSAL LAWS[1]

Do not go where the path may lead, go instead where
there is no path and leave a trail.

— *Ralph Waldo Emerson*

PREAMBLE

Throughout history we have continually been given keys to unlock the doors to a life of happiness. Yet, for some unknown reason, we have thrown away the keys, and accepted society's conditioning that our birth onto this planet was a birth into the school of hard knocks. We were told that life was meant to be a struggle, that there were no free rides. It was about conforming and following the prescribed path. You were required to get an education, enter into the world of work, pay taxes and have a family. Once you had 'done your time', so-to-speak, society would reward you with a golden retirement watch, and off you would go to enjoy your final years in happiness and bliss. Only for some the happiness and bliss didn't really happen. Instead there was illness and loss. Was this what it was all about? Were we only here to struggle through our existence? What would happen if one stepped off the prescribed path to find out just what life was supposed to be about?

---

[1] From *The Book of Ancient Wisdom*, an unpublished manuscript by Beverly D. Blanchard..

~

I grew up in a mixed-ancestry family. My mother was Ojibway and my father was Belorussian-Canadian. Both my parents grew up during the Depression and each had traumatic childhoods. My mother endured the breakup of her family following two painful events, the death of her father followed by abandonment by her mother. All seven children, my mother being the eldest, were either sent to residential school or foster care. My father lost his mother at the age of three and was sent to live with his grandparents in Sturgeon Falls, Ontario. At the age of eleven he was sent back to live with his father and step-mother in Sault Ste. Marie.

My parents met in the logging camps of Regean, Ontario in 1951 and married in 1954. At that time, under the Indian Act of Canada, an Indian woman marrying a white man meant that she lost her status as an Indian and became a Canadian citizen. But this legislation never prevented her from having connections with the reserve. My aunts, uncles and cousins were always a part of our lives. The same was true of my father's Belorussian and Canadian extended families.

My parents were not only of mixed cultures but also from different religious denominations. My father was a non-practicing Protestant and my mother was a devout Catholic. My mother raised all five of her children as Catholic; up until the age of fifteen, I was required to attend church every Sunday. It was at fifteen that I denounced my membership in the church with the proclamation: I am an existentialist. *I do not believe unless I have experienced.* This was met predictably with the comment "she is going through another phase". I didn't quite understand the word existentialist but it did get me out of going to church on Sunday.

After high school I took a year off before attending Laurentian University. When I graduated from University, I initially accepted society's vision for me. I thought happiness would be found in society's prescribed norm of working nine-to-five for the next 35 years of my life. I was not far into this when I realized that it would not bring me happiness. It would actually keep me locked in a life of misery. It was at this time that I developed an insatiable desire to seek out truths about life. I read book after book. I went to workshops. I took up meditation, sensory deprivation and energy work. I immersed myself in First Nations' culture thinking that I would find my answers as to why I was here. Yet, no matter where I turned, I seemed to come to the same conclusion. I needed to step off the beaten path and forge a new path of my own. After much contemplation, I gave up my future security with my government job, and walked. I could no longer work in a job in which I was not living up to my standards. I believed there had to be more to life. Although the road has not always been easy, it was a decision I have never regretted.

After leaving the government, I moved into freelance consulting and split my time between writing reports for clients and searching for more of life's truths. I investigated everything. The problem was that the more I searched, the more confused I became. It seemed everyone had a different definition of truth and a different definition of reality. To the materialists, it was the manifestation of financial and material prosperity: have everything you want at any cost, and define yourself by personal possessions. To the spiritualists, it was the renunciation of financial and material prosperity: have no attachments and define yourself according to poverty. One was living in the world of the haves, and the other was living in the world of the have-nots. Both were too extreme for my liking. Yet both contained some truths about life, and both suggested that people can create their own reality. However, what path was the correct path? Was it the wealth that the materialists had defined as success? Or was it the poverty that spiritualists defined as success? Who was I to believe? What type of reality should one create? In this world in which we live, was it actually possible to create one's own reality? At times, I seemed to be swimming in circles. Each time I thought I found the answers, I would find more questions. Nevertheless, I persevered, and decided that my quest for understanding the truth about life would require effort, devotion and a whole lot of patience. Creating a new reality is not as easy as one might believe.

At points in my search, I seemed be going in the opposite direction of what I thought I was trying to achieve. I wanted financial prosperity, but the rug would be pulled out from under me: I would miss out on a contract, or money I had expected would not materialize. I wanted to create vibrant health, but would injure myself in some way. I wanted to be spiritually enlightened, but would find myself in darkness. It was at these junctures that I would contemplate throwing in the towel on this creating-your-own-reality philosophy. Was it all a big hoax? I would find myself wondering if I had I actually deluded myself into believing I had some control over my life. Perhaps *I* was the one living in an illusion. Sometimes I thought it was all a cosmic joke passed down through the ages and like everything else, no one had ever questioned its validity. In my quest to find myself, perhaps, I had fallen for a scam. Perhaps people just lived and died. That was it. That was all. When faced with these uncertainties, I would force myself to take a step back and review my life to determine if I had actually made some progress. Usually, I discovered some pleasant changes had occurred in me. I gained an understanding of a particular behaviour or an emotion that had sabotaged my efforts. I learned how to relate better with someone or how to let go when the relationship was toxic. At these points I would make some sort of breakthrough. Something would manifest itself. I would find an answer to one of life's questions. Each time I stood at these crossroads, I would realize that there was no fork in the road. For me the path was straight again. I had to persevere.

Then one day it finally dawned on me. It was like a huge light went off. To find happiness, I did not need to accumulate a whole pile of material things. I did not need to become a hermit in the mountains. I did not need to consult with angels or any other outside sources. The truth I was searching for was all within me. All I had to do was accept the fact that happiness was an inside job. I had discovered that although the storm may be raging outside, I had within me a calm center, and it was through this center that I could create my own reality. All I needed to do was find this one point of calmness. This discovery spontaneously changed my feelings to one of happiness.

~

I have put this book together so that you may learn how your inner reality creates your outer reality. It has taken me many years to understand all of this, and I offer you some insights that you may want to consider and which may help you to change your life. What follows are insights into the Universal Laws which govern everyone's life; and if followed will help you to manifest the life you were meant to live.

INTRODUCTION

*Go confidently in the direction of your dreams! Live
the life you've imagined. As you simplify your life, the
laws of the universe will be simpler; solitude will not be
solitude, poverty will not be poverty, nor weakness.*

— Henry David Thoreau

*Twenty years from now you will be more disappointed
by the things that you didn't do than the ones you did
do. So throw off the bowlines. Sail from the safe
harbor. Catch the trade winds in your sails.
Explore. Dream. Discover.*

— Mark Twain

Everyone seems to be talking about how the Law
of Attraction can supply you with continuous joy and
prosperity — a miracle maker. You have only to
identify your wants and desires, write some positive
affirmations that match these wants and desires, and
repeat these affirmations often. Focus! Focus! Focus!
Add emotions. Create pictures in your mind in which
you see yourself as already having achieved your
wants and desires. Finally, take some form of action
towards attaining them. Take these small steps and
you will raise your vibrational level. Miracles will fill
your life. Everything you desire will flow to you.
Money will flow. The shiny red car will appear in the
driveway. You will meet your soulmate. Life will be
filled with continuous, unending happiness and bliss.

Will it really? It all sounds simple and easy. The
reality is however, that the Law of Attraction alone

will not bring you the success or happiness you desire by simply engaging in those simple techniques. I am not saying that the Law of Attraction does not exist or does not work. It does work. There is a Law of Attraction operating in our Universe; however, this law requires a significant amount of work on your inner self. It requires commitment and sometimes a lot of patience. It will never work if you utilize the Law of Attraction with the intent of fulfilling all your desires. Think what life would be if you got everything you thought you desired! Think back to a time when you were angry. Did you really want those desires, born of anger, to come true? Besides, getting everything you desire all at once is not something that is feasible. Life is about enjoying the journey. It is not about continually craving new desires. For once fulfilled, there must always be another desire and another goal. Round and round the circle you go, and life becomes filled with only fleeting moments of happiness; you get what you want — elation followed by depression. If you are not centered in yourself, being wealthy and having all the material things life has to offer means that happiness can still elude you. If happiness was defined by money and material goods, many of the world celebrities would not be entering 'rehab' to deal with their alcohol and drug addictions, depression or weight problems. They would not be attempting to fill up their lives with outside commodities, friends and hangers-on. Happiness has to begin from the inside. Only then can material acquisitions become bonuses of life.

The Law of Attraction also includes a whole set of other laws which prevail in this Universe. It is important to understand that all the laws cannot be distilled into "monitoring your thoughts and feelings". None of these laws, including the Law of Attraction, operate in isolation. When you are thinking of changing your life it is important to be aware of this. If you are not aware of the whole system, and you chose to only work within the confines of the Law of Attraction, you will be frustrated and disappointed. Your journey through this life is not only about accumulating material goods and/or money. Material possessions are good, but they are not the whole goal. They are a means to getting you to where you need to go on your journey of growth, and the journey of growth is not about getting power, prestige, and money or fulfilling all your passions and desires. It is about operating from your calm inner being even when life is spinning around you like a tornado. It is also about spontaneity. It is learning to read the signals of life, and going with the flow.

An important consideration with regards to the Universal Laws (the Laws of Life) is that they have been operating since the beginning time. How you go through this life depends on your understanding of them. Operate with them, and your life flows like a river. Operate against them, and it is like swimming up-stream. Your life will be filled with frustration in which you will continually feel that you are at the mercy of some outside force. *If only* and *I will* are mantras filling that void inside you. The Law of Attraction is only one aspect of a whole reality, and for you to successfully change your life, you need to become aware of the other laws.

It is also important to understand that changing your life requires work and reprogramming. You came into this world a clean slate. Unfortunately, it has not stayed that way. Through the course of your life, your parents, the environment you live in, and society has filled you with a lot of programs which have been running the show. It is these programs that are keeping you from moving with the flow of life. Rightly or wrongly, they have provided you with limitations; limitations which are really your beliefs. In order to change your life, sometimes you have to dig deep and really understand why you are so heavily rooted in a particular belief. Once you have fully understood it, then you can transform it.

Once you get moving on your journey of change, you may find that the things you thought would bring you happiness, like money, society's acceptance or parental approval, are no longer important to you. You may find that moving through the world in a balanced and peaceful manner will have more significance for you. You may discover that the true goal in life is not growing old but growing upwards and gaining wisdom. It is about understanding that material attachments, academic achievements, power and prestige are not the factors which define the real you. There is nothing intrinsically bad about any of these things; however, when you die the money, house, car, career and whatever it is that you have acquired, cannot be taken with you. When you leave this earth, the only thing that leaves with you is your inner being. Did you become wise or did you just accumulate stuff? Did you discover that the goal of life was to experience life? Or did you spend your life running after the goal of making a living, living up to society's expectations? Did you live a life seeking approval? Life is not about dragging yourself to the grave. It is about enjoying every moment while you are here.

The very first thing that you must understand when working with the Universal Laws is that everything and everyone is really just energy vibrating at different frequencies. Accept the fact that you are energy vibrating in human form, and decide how you will work with this energy. Your peace, happiness and success are not dependent on outside circumstances. It is not dependent on whether others accept you or do not accept you. It is not about the family you were born into, or the country you reside in. It is not about the color of your skin, or the culture in which you were raised. Your happiness is totally dependent upon you. You have been given a body and how you go through life is totally up to you. You can see everything happening in your life as a struggle or you can undertake the journey of life joyously, seeing everything that happens to you as a simple opportunity to learn and grow upwards. There are no mistakes. There are no grades. There is no need for anyone else's approval. There is no one standing over you in judgment. Life is just simply a series of experiences, and through these experiences you are offered the opportunity to grow in understanding.

These Laws are somewhat like life's Operating Guide. In working with them you will learn to understand that in life there really are no choices. There is just life, and life is love. Life is what is happening to you in the moment. Add choice into the equation and you break the flow. You must be spontaneous in your life. If you are operating from true love, your actions are in accordance with your intention. Past experiences should not cloud your present moment. You learn how to respond to life's experiences. When you respond to something you are operating in the *now*. When you react to something you are operating from your memory and the accumulation of the detritus of the past. The more you respond, the more happiness flows in your life. Through working with all the Universal Laws, you can learn to see each moment either as new or as a re-enactment of your past experiences. There really is no choice.

Before I begin outlining some of the different Universal Laws and how you can work with them to bring about change in your life, it is important to understand that there really is no hierarchical structure to the Universal Laws - one is not more important than another. They work in unison, and are not necessarily mutually exclusive. Some laws do work better in conjunction with other laws. This is one of the main reasons why some people never achieve their goals under the Law of Attraction alone; the world does not operate solely according to our wishes and desires. The Universal Laws will enhance your opportunities, helping you flow along with life instead of against life. You create a life instead of haphazardly accepting what life brings to you.

Universal Laws are an extension of the Creator/God/Great Spirit/Source Energy/Universe/Existence or whatever you want to call the originator. For the purposes of this book, I will use many of these terms interchangeably. It is important however to understand, that when I use the word 'God', I am not talking about a man sitting up in the sky who is controlling everything and determining whose prayers he shall answer. I am referring to God as the ultimate energy source to which we are all connected. God is in everything and everything is in God. Anything that is living is filled with that energy, and the Universal Laws are this energy in action. These laws apply all the time to everyone and everywhere. They are part of the whole and the easiest way to view them in operation is to look at nature.

The following are some of the Laws that I speak about in the *Book of Ancient Wisdom*. Here I have only highlighted the ones which I feel can assist you on your journey. I have included exercises for each of the laws which will help you to make life changes. While you may understand these laws intellectually, practice will increase their benefit to you. If the exercise does not appear to work for you, try something else. Recognize that within these laws, there is no good or bad, right or wrong. There is no such thing as moral judgments; moral judgments are manmade. The more you become aware of these laws, the more they will work for you. Let these laws guide your living and you will flow through life. There will be days when you feel lost in the valley of darkness, but you will be able to handle yourself differently, and in time will find yourself there less often. Instead of getting bent out of shape when life throws you challenges, you will adapt and change. Go with the flow. Is this not what life is all about?

THE LAW OF ONE

*A person experiences life as something separated from
the rest - a kind of optical delusion of consciousness.
Our task must be to free ourselves from this self-
imposed prison, and through compassion, to find the
reality of Oneness.*

— Albert Einstein

*A miracle is nothing more or less than this. Anyone
who has come into knowledge of his true identity, of
his oneness with the all-pervading wisdom and power,
this makes it possible for laws higher than the
ordinary mind knows of to be revealed to him.*

— Ralph Waldo Emerson

The Law of One simply states that we are all related
and connected. There is one source and everything is
contained within the whole. I am you and you are
me. We may be unique beings but we are not separated
beings. There is no separation in the world, and every-
thing you think, do and say has an effect on the world
around you. Everything and everyone is contained
within this sphere. Many indigenous populations have
demonstrated this type of understanding in their
philosophy on life. They believe everything and every-
one is related, and that everything contained within
the circle of Existence, is their family. When they pray,
they give thanks to the Great Spirit, Grandfather Sun,
Grandmother Moon, Father Sky, Mother Earth, the
winged, the four-legged, the two-legged and the four
elements. Everyone is seen as a part of the Great Spirit's

family, and they recognize that everything and everyone is contained within the whole. Everything has a purpose. There was no division or boundaries since no one holds or possesses property.

To understand this law on a personal level, you need only look at your own body. To the eye the body's boundary is the skin which keeps everything together. Within the skin there are various organs and glands, muscles, connective tissues, energy centers and a blood supply comprised of billions of cells. Although each part of you has a specific function and looks to be separate, they are actually all connected and working within the whole of you.

To further the analogy, look at the connection between humans and trees. In order to survive, human beings breathe in oxygen and exhale carbon dioxide. Trees on the other hand, breathe in carbon dioxide and exhale oxygen to survive. Without the trees, where would man be? Everything within and around you is connected. Everything is energy spinning in form.

Under the Law of One, you and God are one. No one is more special than anyone else. Everyone and everything is a spark of the original source energy. Everyone is equal, and there is no higher or lower. There is only one. Once you accept this concept, it changes the context in which you experience everything in your life - past, present and future. You realize the individual that is you does not represent the totality of God. It only represents a spark of the whole. However, without your spark there is no whole. All the other laws are contained within this law.

EXERCISES

1. See everything and everyone as energy in action. As you go about your day, mentally visualize everyone as God. Mentally say to yourself, There is God /Universal Light Source /the Great Spirit. to everyone and every living thing you see around you. You see someone picking trash out of a container mentally say *There is God picking trash out of a container.* Someone is running for the bus, *There is God running for the bus.* You see a bird flying in the air, *There is God flying in the air.* A tree swaying in wind, *There is God swaying in the wind.* As you walk into your office and you see your co-worker at her desk, *There is God working at her desk.* Practice these affirmations for the next seven days.

2. See everything and everyone as you-in-action. As you go about your day, visualize everyone as you. Say to yourself, *There I go.* to everyone and every living thing you see around you. You see someone picking trash out of a container mentally say, *There I go picking trash out of a container.* Someone is running for the bus, *There I go running for the bus.* You see a bird flying in the air, *There I go flying in the air.* A tree swaying in wind, *There I go swaying in the wind.* As you walk into your office and you see your co-worker at her desk, *There I am working at my desk.* Practice these affirmations for the next seven days.

3. Release yourself from the concept of *I,*
mine and *my*. Once you use the words *I, mine*
and *my,* you make yourself separate from
everyone and everything. Try removing the
words *I, mine* and *my* from your vocabulary
for a week. Instead of saying, *I am going to*
work say, *We are going to work.* Instead of saying,
I am going to my house say, *We are going to our*
house.

LAW OF ABUNDANCE

Unblest is he who thinks himself unblest.

— *Seneca*

But what shall it profit a man if he shall gain the whole and lose his own soul.

— *Mark 8:36*

The Law of Abundance teaches that there is no need for miserly conduct. There is no need to operate with greed. There is nothing to fear. Give freely and do not hoard. There is always enough for everyone. There is enough food, water, energy and resources on this planet for everyone. This does not mean however that we should squander our resources and operate in a careless fashion. The Law of Abundance states that our needs will be supplied. The Universe is continually growing, producing and thriving. To see the Law of Abundance in action, you need only look at nature. Does a bird worry whether it is going to have enough material to build its nest? Watch as they build their nests; they do not complain about the lack of branches. Neither do squirrels seem to worry about whether they will have enough nuts for winter. Apple trees produce an abundance of apples from their branches and with more than enough fallen on the ground to be enjoyed by the many creatures that dwell below. Everything works in such a way that universal needs are met.

Although politicians, economists and environmentalists would have us believe that we live on a planet of scarcity, nothing could be further from the truth. Mother Earth has an infinite amount of resources and these resources will be there as we need them. History has proven this. For instance, during the 1800s there was a dependency upon whale oil, and it was predicted that the whale supply would run out. It was at this point that man created the automobile, and fossil fuels were discovered to meet the needs of this new technology. Man's discovery of electricity moved us away from oil burning lamps. Man has always discovered new technologies when he needed them. As we move forward into the future, alternative sources of energy will be found to replace the dependency on fossil fuels or new sources of fossil fuels will be discovered. The illusion of scarcity in our society is enhanced by the manmade boundaries that we have established to construct nations and through our economic models. These models are purely based on fear and greed. Recognize that there is no scarcity of resources but that there exists rather a scarcity in cooperation amongst mankind.

EXERCISES (ABBUNDANCE)

1. Look at your life and see the abundance you already have. Do you have your health? A roof over your head? A loving spouse/partner? Food in the refrigerator? Clean water? Make a list of everything that you have in your life, and turn away from scarcity-based thinking. You have abundance. Accept it. Live your life.

2. If you think you are experiencing shortages, think again. The Universe may be trying to supply you with what you need but you may be turning down the gifts. Ask yourself: *Where or what am I resisting in my life? When am I saying no? What would I do if I had no fear, no shame?*

3. Manufactured fear or true fear. Scarcity-based thinking is very much based on manufactured fear. Manufactured fear has its roots in the fear-based concept that *I will not get my share.* This belief is usually strengthened through worry about possible scenarios in an imaginary future. Most people in society are operating on the manufactured fear model. True fear on the other hand is our body's warning mechanism. It is the fight or flight mechanism which is used for survival. Throughout the day take the time to ask yourself: Is this situation real or am I manufacturing fear? If you are manufacturing fear, you are wasting precious energy.

LAW OF ATTRACTION

A wise man makes his own decisions; an ignorant man follows public opinion.

— *Chinese Proverb*

The Law of Attraction demonstrates how we create the things, events and people that come into our lives. Our thoughts, feelings, words and actions produce energies which attract like energies. Negative energies attract negative experiences and positive energies attract positive experiences.

Most people go through life identifying what it is that they do *not* want in life. They do *not* want to date any more losers. They do not want to be in a dead-end relationship or career. They do not want to be sick anymore. *I do not want* becomes their mantra. They have identified what they don't want and they just keep replaying it. Without realizing it, they focus on the negative and are actually attracting more of the things they do not want in their life; they date more losers, and have another dead-end relationship. Take the time to understand this simple little fact about how the mind works. It is only your conscious mind which has the ability to distinguish between a positive and negative word. Your subconscious mind, on the other hand, does not process or integrate negative words. Words such as *no, not, never* go directly into the subconscious as though they were positive and may be one of the reasons why many people continue to have frustrating lives. By identifying with what they do not want, they do not identify what they do want.

For the Law of Attraction to work you must be aware of what it is that you are thinking and saying to yourself and to others at all times. Nothing escapes this law; you cannot lie on any level. If you mentally affirm that you are prosperous one minute and in the next tell someone that you are always broke, then your positive affirmation will be cancelled by the negative. Positive affirmations are only good if you are consistent on all levels of your life, including your thoughts and words. Your thoughts and words are energy and it is through these venues that you manifest what it is you want in your life.

When you initially start working with the Law of Attraction, you may want to create your own wish-list using the words, *I prefer* instead of the words *I want* or *I desire*. *I prefer* helps to keep you consistently positive because it provides you with a mechanism to avoid disappointment. Sometimes the Universe operates according to a schedule different than what you would like. Or sometimes, what you are trying to manifest is something that is not in your best interests. You may think you want it, but on a subconscious level you may not want it at all. It is at these times that you have to be vigilant to keep yourself positive. Reverting back to negative thinking and behaviors will lower your vibrational level and attract what you give out.

EXERCISES

1. What is it you that you do not want in your life? Make a list of all the things, situations and things you do not want in your life. After you are finished, burn it, rip it to pieces, or toss it in the garbage. Now make a list of all the things you would prefer in your life. Focus only on this list.

2. Change the way you speak. If you find yourself constantly saying, *I don't want...* get into the habit of stopping yourself. Consciously say, *I cancel that manifestation. Here is what I do prefer...* You can be even more dramatic and wave your arms in the air and say, *Canceling! Canceling! Canceling! Canceling that manifestation!* when you use the words, *I don't want...*

3. The hungry ghost. Sometimes we keep buying or desiring things in hopes that they will fill a void within us and bring us happiness. We keep looking in the refrigerator even though we are not hungry. We go on shopping sprees even though we have 200 pairs of black pants in our closet. We consume alcohol and drugs to combat boredom. We spend our life compensating through consumption in an effort to fill a void. The problem is consumption does not make us feel any better. If you are continually consuming for the sake of filling yourself up, you need to take a time-out and ask yourself, what is it you truly desire? What exactly do you prefer in your life?

(ATTRACTION)

4. Go on a *negativity* diet. Reduce your use of negative thinking. You are what you focus on, whether it is negative or positive. Look only for the good and positive in everything.

LAW OF
CAUSE AND EFFECT

*There are two things to aim at in life; first, to get what
you want; and, after that, to enjoy it. Only the wisest
of mankind achieve the second.*
— *Logan Pearsall Smith*

Under the Law of Cause and Effect everything
you do in this world has a reaction and for every action
there must be an equal and opposite reaction. Drop a
pebble in a pond and it ripples outward and creates an
effect. There is nothing in this Universe that happens
by chance or happenstance. Every action has a reaction
or consequence, and sometimes these reactions are
far reaching. You chew out one of your employees;
the employee goes home and chews out their spouse;
that spouse may chew out one of the children; the child
chews out one of their friends. Everything you do
ripples outward and has an effect. Every thought, word,
feeling and action you have or say is energy and it is
that energy that creates an effect in this world.

On a personal level, what you think about most often
is what you will end up getting. Change your thinking
and you change your life. Your thinking is creating the
experiences you get. *But wait*, you say, *I do not want all this
crap that keeps coming at me. I keep thinking good thoughts.* Are
you really? Do you wake up on a rainy Monday
morning and tell yourself, this is going to be another
miserable week? Do you tell yourself that you never
have enough time and money to do what you want?
Do you look at the general socio-economic conditions
and tell yourself that it is impossible to realize your
potential? Do you say: *I am too sick; I am too fat; I do not*

105

know the right people; This world is a horrid place. Simple cure: just stop, stop saying those things.

If something in your life is not working the way you want, it is important to understand that somewhere or sometime there was a thought, word or deed that caused a wave of undesirable energy. To re-balance and calm this energy requires that you change your thoughts, words and deeds into a more positive direction. Initially it is difficult to do; old habits are hard to break. We start out wonderfully the first week and then something happens that throws us back on the negativity trail. You have to keep at it and break the old programming. One of the fastest ways to do this is to change your words, thoughts and deeds to ones that involve unconditional love, forgiveness and compassion. What you have today is a result of the sowing you did in the past. What you will have tomorrow is what you are sowing today. Release the past. It is dead. Start sowing the seeds that contain positive and loving thoughts from this present moment, and the next present moment, and the next. Life is not stagnant and each moment is new. In life, nothing is ever repeated exactly the same way.

Equally important as the words you use, are the actions you take. Talk can be cheap. *Tomorrow I am going to be more positive; tomorrow I am going to lose weight.* There is no action in these statements. Just talking about losing weight is not going to change your weight. You have to implement the actions necessary to lose the weight the moment you make the statement. The thought is there to assist you, but it alone will not change much in your life. Think about how many thoughts you have. Action is the one of the most important aspects in the whole process of im-plementing change in your life. Do everything now.

EXERCISES

1. Tune in to your internal dialogue. We all talk to ourselves and you may be very surprised to discover that your constant internal chatter can often be your own worst enemy. How often have you called yourself stupid, an idiot or had a morning conversation with yourself planning the argument you were going to have with your boss. Spend a few days listening to your internal dialogue and seek to change the patterns that are not working for you. You can even tell yourself to shut up once in awhile.

2. Remove the words: 'should', 'cannot', 'have not', 'but' and 'I will become' from your vocabulary. There is nothing wrong with these words. You just have to understand the context of how you are using them. How many times have you said to someone: *I just can't do it?* Only you really meant, *I really don't want to do it.* Does the word 'should' conjure up your parent's voice when you did something wrong? *You should have done it this or that way.* The words 'have not' implies lack. 'But' is a frequently used word that tends to discount anything positive previously said. For example, *I lost ten pounds, but I will probably gain it back.* The positive has been offset by the negative.

(CAUSE AND EFFECT)

3. After you have spent some time identifying your thoughts and words, go to the root cause of why you are relearning the same old lessons. What is the underlying behaviour that is not allowing you to achieve your preference? Thoughts and words are just the symptoms. What is at the root? Once you understand the root, the change proceeds.

LAW OF COMPASSION

You must get your living by loving.

— Henry David Thoreau

Lord let me not judge a man until I have walked two moons in his moccasins.

— Navajo Prayer

The Law of Compassion is allowing tenderness and kindness into all your thoughts and actions with yourself and others. It is about softening your attitude, and allowing others to be who they are without judgments or condemnation. Under the Law of Compassion one simply recognizes that everyone, including you, is not perfect and that we all operate in accordance with our own set of beliefs, conditioning and capabilities. Compassion does not mean that you have to change your stance or even agree with what the other person or group is saying or doing. You simply allow yourself to see the world through someone else's eyes. The observer becomes the observed.

To be compassionate you have to begin with you. If you cannot offer yourself understanding, forgiveness and loving kindness you can never give genuine compassion to someone else. The first step in compassion is releasing all judgments and condemnations about yourself and others. In the outer world see everyone as your teacher. Each one is providing you with the gift of experience. How you go through that experience is up to you. You are responsible for your part in the relationship. Your responsibility lies in your reaction

109

which is usually based on a past experience. Someone insults you and immediately you go on the defensive and yet, if someone flatters you your ego swells. There are some situations that do require one to go on the defensive but operating from past experience has become most people's strategy for living. Instead of dealing with life as it arises they swallow their anger and resentment where it festers. Every experience becomes a series of habitual reactions repeated throughout your lifetime. Until one day you blow. Swallowing anger and resentment and trying to be compassionate is not the same as being truly compassionate. Doing anything with an ounce of anger and resentment is not compassion. No matter what has been done to you, harbor no ill feelings because if you harbor hatred and anger it will only eat away at you like a cancer. Offer forgiveness and recognize that you may have done things in your life in which your own behavior was less than stellar. Also recognize that some of the most difficult people and situations usually provide you with opportunities for growth.

Compassion is not about sympathy, empathy or pity. It is not about doing something out of politeness, obligation or guilt. Living a compassionate life does not mean being a doormat to others. It does not mean allowing others to dump all their problems on you or to take advantage of you. To do any of this means you are not operating out of compassion. Living a compassionate life is about truly listening and taking the time to understand someone else's situation or circumstances. Move through the world with compassion, and the world will present you with unique gifts.

EXERCISES

1. Open your heart. Talk to someone you do not know. You get on the same bus or walk the same route everyday and pass the same people everyday. Take the time to talk to these people and find out about them. Take the time to really listen. They may even be the person who offers you a piece of advice that sets you on a different path.

2. Walk in someone else's moccasins. Next time you feel that someone has done something that you perceive as wrong, before you verbally attack them, pause and take a step in their shoes. Try to understand what may be motivating them. For most people you may find that either it is an expression of love or a call for love. Recognize that it is far easier to forgive someone when you have taken the time to understand what motivates their behavior. To get in the habit of walking in someone else's shoes, next time you are walking behind someone step into their footsteps. Follow them and let yourself become them.

3. Think back to a time when you were able to be yourself. How did you feel? Hold that feeling. Keep holding that feeling. Keep holding it.

4. Think back to a time when you were not paid attention to. How did you feel? Go to the root of this feeling. What did you really fear? Was it real? Or were you manufacturing it?

LAW OF COMPENSATION

Do not invite rich people to your house for dinner. You will be repaid by their inviting you to their house for dinner. Invite poor people to your house for dinner. They cannot repay you, so the universe must repay you.

— *Khalil Gibran*

This Universal Law is the Law of Cause and Effect applied to the blessings and abundance that are provided for you. The visible effects of your actions are given to you in gifts, money, inheritances, friendships, and blessings. You will receive just remuneration based on your actions; give out good and it flows back to you; give out crap and *it* flows back to you. What goes around comes around. One word of caution, you must give from your heart with no expectation of return.

Too often I hear people saying, *I do good things. I help people out and yet nothing good comes of it.* Are you really acting with kindness? Are you really giving for the sheer joy of giving? Or are you giving out from some form of obligation or guilt? Are you giving to gain other people's approval? Are you giving because you want other people to see you as good? Are you giving because you want a tax break? Are you giving out of pity? If you are giving for any of these reasons you are not truly giving. You are operating under a façade. Your giving is tied to your head and not to your heart. Give from the heart and give freely with no expectation of receiving and you will open the floodgates to receive that which is truly yours.

EXERCISES

1. Become aware of the action, not the result. Practice outrageous acts of kindness. Put some money in someone's expired parking meter. Smile at people as you move through your day. Give some money to someone who looks like they need it — or even to someone who doesn't need it. Buy the person in the line behind you a coffee.

2. Write out the things that you are doing in order to get something back from others, and then stop doing them. Doing anything from the perspective of obligation only ferments resentment inside you.

3. If someone asks you to do something or give money to a charity and you do not really want to, say *no*. Stop giving from guilt and obligations. Instead of giving in money, make your everyday interactions an act of kindness.

LAW OF CONSCIOUS DETACHMENT

*Drop the question what tomorrow may bring, and
count as profit every day that fate allows you.*
— *Horace*

Also known as the Law of Allowing, this Universal Law means that when you accept what is, and release yourself from the attachment of trying to make things go your way, something always clicks for you. For it is at the point of release that the universe opens up to you and provides you with opportunities and solutions. More simply, if something you are trying to manifest is not happening, it is sometimes better to step away and forget about it for a while. Perhaps you are trying too hard, and by focusing on trying, are missing the obvious. Many of the great scientists worked with this law. Einstein spent hours in the bathtub and it was said that some of his greatest ideas came when he was in that bath relaxing and playing with bubbles. You cannot push the river and you cannot speed some things up. Everything happens in its own time, and sometimes you just have to let go and trust that the answers or experiences will come to you. At other times, it may mean that the goal you are so focused on is not in your best interests. It may never happen. To continue pushing will only bring frustration and misery. All you need to do is to let go of all possible outcomes. Do something else. Let loose and let go. Surrender it over to the Universe. Trust that what is yours will come to you.

EXERCISES

1. Divert your attention. Go for a walk. Take a bath. Date someone else. Work on something else but move your attention away from whatever it is that you think you want.

2. Give up the spiritual temper tantrums. Getting angry will not make things happen faster; in fact it will interfere with your manifestation by demonstrating that you are feeling frustrated. You need to maintain a positive vibration while you are also consciously detaching from whatever it is you want.

Into The Waves

REFLECTIONS

1. YOUR STORY

Contrary to what you may have been taught, life is not meant to be a struggle. You are neither a victim of circumstance nor happenstance. You are not without power. Life is a journey of experiences that you have created for yourself. If you find you are living in some form of misery, it is because you have arrived there through your own thoughts, beliefs, superstitions and conditioning. Accept that you are responsible for everything in your life. Own your life and, if you don't like how things are going, make the decision to write yourself a new story. It is in the writing of the new story that you claim your power.

2. THE NOW

In life there is no time like now. Psychological change happens in the *Now* where there is no time. Most physical change, movement or learning usually happens through time. To change the psychological, you need to make a decision to reach for a higher-feeling thought. Recognize that every moment creates the next moment. Regardless of circumstances, it is in the moment that you get to chose how you want to feel. Choose carefully. Check in often with yourself and ask: How am I doing now? Am I feeling the way I want to feel?

3. ATTRACTION

In life you get what you give. Give love; you get love back. Tell lies and you will be lied to. Cheat someone and you shall be cheated. Miserable people attract miserable people. Like attracts like and it is your vibration that brings experiences to you. Everything that happens to you happens because of you and you are never without the power to change your life. Don't like the people, places or situations in your life? Take a look within at what you are thinking. Look at your own actions. Are you spending your life complaining about what's wrong? Beat the drum of what's wrong in your life or in your world and you open the door to more negativity. Focus only on what you want; not on where you are. Begin now. The inner is always the starting point for change.

4. SILENCE

Make room for silence on a daily basis. The mind has an incessant need to chatter about useless and irrelevant topics and will always lead you astray. The mind is your servant and it must be controlled. Don't let your mind be your master. Learn to take time to still your thoughts; over-thinking is wasted energy. Practice meditation and focus on your breathing. Take control and listen to your inner guidance. All solutions are found in silence.

5. LOVE

In life there really is only one choice and that choice is love. The opposite of love is not hate. There is no opposite of love. If you are living a life of *bona fide* love then there is no conflict. It is only in conflict that you need choices. With choice, discord is created and love never lives in discord. Love is love. There is no conflict when you live through love. Love has no conditions. There are no strings. To give love with conditions turns it into a business transaction; an ugly tit-for-tat contract in which there is an accounting of each *love* transaction. Accept that love is like a flower. It cares not who smells its fragrance. It just fills the air. Love even loves those who are unlovable.

6. IDEALS

Life is not about creating ideals or living a life based on past traditions and rituals. All ideals are rooted in past memories and lead to repetition. A life of repetitions is not a life. Toss customs and traditions out the window for they bind you to a past that is dead and teaches you to distrust your own innate knowing. Creation is found only in the spontaneous, the innocent, with no preconceived notions.

7. INNER SPACE

Do not wait to learn that greatness lives within you. It cannot be found in outside sources. It cannot be measured by the number of awards or certificates you have on your wall. Never bow down to outside authority and recognize that other people's opinions are irrelevant and that experts may not necessarily be expert. Play your role in life strong and whole. Magnificence lies within. Find it and tap into it. Accept it into your life and great changes will happen.

8. THE PAST

Never look back. The past only tethers you to unnecessary attachments and emotions. It fosters regret, doubt and guilt. It robs you of the moment. Release yourself from the past. What has happened has happened. You cannot change it. There is no reason to defend, justify or explain who you are and why you are here. Let it go and make feeling good in the present moment the only thing that matters.

9. CONFORMITY

Release yourself from the game of conformity. It is not worth playing. There is no security in the mob and if you follow groupthink it will only lead you away from your own inner intelligence. You are a unique being. Accept yourself and be proud of who you are. Listen only to the stirrings of your heart and allow them to guide you. Your inner source is the only guidance you can trust.

10. LAUGHTER

Lighten up. Being serious is detrimental to your well-being. It wears you down and creates undue stress in your life. Your mood can be changed instantly by smiling and laughing. Being serious is for the fools who have been taught that there is no enjoyment in life. These are the individuals who postpone living and day-by-day drag themselves to the grave. What good is life if you have not lived?

11. CONSISTENCY

Don't take comfort in consistency. Life is not stagnant; everything changes. Your friends today may be your enemies tomorrow and vice-versa. One day you have a job and the next day you are unemployed. Someone you love may leave you. Appreciate the moments in your life and recognize the only consistency is your connection to your inner being.

12. ACTION

Words have no meaning. Judge others on their actions for it is their actions that speak louder than words. There are many in this world that will use flowery words to cover up their ill intent. In your desire to be liked do not allow yourself to fall victim to the flattery heaped upon you by others. These individuals will influence you in ways contrary to your best interests.

13. SOURCE ENERGY

Your emotions indicate whether you are aligned with your inner source or not. Your inner source will never join you in a pity party. If you find yourself experiencing boredom, sadness, frustration or anger, recognize that these are indicators that you are not aligned with your source energy. To realign with your inner source take your focus away from the issue that is consuming your current state of mind. Watch a funny movie. Read an interesting book. Take a walk. Meditate. Do anything that allows you to reconnect with your source energy.

14. GOODNESS

Try to give people the benefit of the doubt. Regardless of outside appearances many people in this world are really scared little children operating under an adult façade. Your inner being only sees the good in others. Do your best to see the good in others and all things. When you do, it will magnify their goodness and you will allow them to connect to their own inner source.

END

INDEX

ABOUT THE AUTHOR

Beverly Diana Blanchard is an Ojibway First Nation from Northern Ontario. She holds a degree in Economics from Laurentian University. A former Public Servant, she has been a consultant to First Nation and Inuit organizations on a variety of issues. Using the wisdom of Indigenous tribal cultures and ancient spiritual traditions as the foundation of her writing and workshops, she focuses on enabling people to explore, enjoy and embrace life.

Beverly is a writer and personal development coach based in Sault Ste. Marie and Ottawa, Canada.

ABOUT THE ILLUSTRATIONS

The *Eagle* sketch, and the drawing *We are One, We are all Unique* (p. 62) are by Beverly. The art work *Quilt* was completed by her talented niece Eryn, a First Nation Ojibway, at the age of eight (p. ii and the circles throughout).